Safety Training for Obstetric Emergencies

The OB F.A.S.T Approach

GIANCARLO MARI, M.D., M.B.A., F.A.C.O.G., F.A.I.U.M., F.A.G.O.S.

Professor and Chairman
Department of Obstetrics and Gynecology
The University of Tennessee Health Science Center
Memphis, TN, United States

ELSEVIER

Notices

Publisher: Meloni Dolores
Acquisition Editor: Sarah Barth
Editorial Project Manager: Pat Gonzalez
Production Project Manager: Kiruthika Govindaraju
Cover Designer: Alan Studholme

3251 Riverport Lane
St. Louis, Missouri 63043

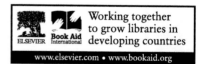

Working together
to grow libraries in
developing countries

www.elsevier.com • www.bookaid.org

In memory of my parents and for Laura, Michael, and Camilla.

List of Contributors

Pedro Argoti, MD
Assistant Professor
Ultrasound Fellow
Department of Obstetrics and Gynecology
UTHSC
Memphis, TN, United States

Jennifer Barr, MD
Fellow
Maternal Fetal Medicine
Department of Obstetrics and Gynecology
UTHSC
Memphis, TN, United States

Jennifer Carelle, MSHS, RDM, RVT, RT(R)
Sonographer Coordinator
Maternal Fetal Medicine
Departments of Obstetrics and Gynecology
UTHSC
Memphis, TN, United States

Sandeep ChilaKala, MD
Assistant Professor
Neonatology Division
Department of Pediatrics
UTHSC
Memphis, TN, United States

Ravprest Gill, MD
Department of Anesthesia
Baptist Medical Center
Memphis, TN, United States

Karen Hamilton, BSN, RN
IT Senior Clinical Analyst
Regional One Health
Memphis, TN, United States

Genxia Li, MD
The Third Affiliated Hospital of
    Zhengzhou University
Maternal and Child Health Hospital of
    Henan Province
Zhengzhou City, Henan Province, China

Bonnie Miller, BSN, RN
Clinical Nurse Specialist for Women's
    Health and Neonatology
Regional One Health
Memphis, TN, United States

Francesco Napoleone, MD
Research Fellow
Department of Obstetrics and Gynecology
UTHSC
Memphis, TN, United States

Mauro Schenone, MD
Associate Professor
Director Maternal Fetal Medicine Division
Department of Obstetrics and Gynecology
UTHSC
Memphis, TN, United States

Danielle Tate, MD
Assistant Professor
Director of the High Risk Clinic
Maternal Fetal Medicine
Department of Obstetrics and Gynecology
UTHSC
Memphis, TN, United States

A Brief History of the Obstetrics Simulation Program at the University of Tennessee Health Science Center and Regional One Health, Memphis

When I was a resident in obstetrics and gynecology (ob/gyn), we used to rotate in one hospital where the second-year resident was on the labor and delivery (L&D) suite at night alone, or with only one medical student. The attending physician was on call at home. In an emergency, he/she had to reach the hospital within 30 minutes. The resident on duty applied forceps and performed cesarean deliveries with the student as assistant or with the surgery residents. Although we had a baby mannequin and a pelvis simulator in our L&D suite that we used to review the steps for vaginal delivery, there was not a big emphasis on simulation. The older obstetricians would learn on the patients. One of my senior residents related his learning experience in the application of the Kielland forceps: the attending applied the forceps, rotated the fetal head from transverse to occiput anterior, rotated the head back in the transverse presentation, removed the forceps, and then invited the resident to apply it again. This learning was the old obstetrics. However, other areas of medicine were similar. I remember ob/gyn interns applying Swan–Ganz catheters without direct supervision during their rotation in the Surgical Intensive Care Unit.

I have practiced obstetrics and gynecology in three different continents (Europe, America, and Asia) and I can state that in many areas of the world, obstetricians who never received a full training and have learned on the field continue to perform unnecessary and risky procedures with consequences for mothers and their babies. Most of the time, the outcome will still be good because, even without any intervention, patients are able to physiologically deliver their babies. For high-risk pregnancies, however, training is fundamental. It is disheartening to hear what happens when the team is not prepared, and intervention causes more harm than good.

The following case, which occurred in one small hospital, is an example:

A healthy 36-year-old patient presents in labor at 39 weeks' gestation. Her labor progresses normally during the night. Her obstetrician, who has been in practice for more than 30 years, is at home and does not inquire about his patient during the night. In the morning he goes to the hospital and finds his patient in the delivery room, fully dilated. He loudly asks why he has not been called during the night. A vacuum application is then performed because, the patient is told, there is "uterine atony," but the application fails. Subsequently, she undergoes a cesarean delivery via Pfannenstiel incision and delivers a 6 lb 6 oz infant. The mother must wait 4 hours following the delivery before she can see her baby. The baby pictures reviewed by an expert suggest that the vacuum had not been applied appropriately.

Two days following the cesarean section, the mother develops an "ileus" and she is told that her baby is doing well. One hour later she is informed that her baby is having focal seizures of the right extremities, and he needs to be transferred to another facility. One hour after that, the patient is informed that she has to be transferred to another facility as well, because the physicians at her current hospital do not feel comfortable managing her. The obstetrician justifies the transfers saying that the doctors of that hospital could not be trusted. The result is that the patient and her baby are transferred to two different facilities in two different cities. A few hours following the transfer, the patient undergoes a puboxyphoid laparotomy following an abdominal X-ray confirming an ileus. When the family requests a second opinion, the obstetrician says that it is too late and he performs the laparotomy with a general surgeon. At surgery, the bowel is pink and normal, slightly distended. Two small peritoneal adhesions are found and the doctors justify the necessity of the surgery because of those adhesions. The patient is kept in the hospital for 10 more days as her postoperative period is complicated by fever on day six. She complains of urinary burning but she is not started on antibiotics for urinary infection, caused by the prolonged indwelling Foley catheter, until day nine. The patient rarely sees her obstetrician during the hospital stay and at discharge she is told to see a surgeon in her town.

A cerebral MRI performed on the infant 6 weeks after delivery suggests that there was cerebral bleeding and hypoxia at the time of delivery.

This case emphasizes several important aspects that will be discussed in this book: communication, teamwork, technical and non-technical skills. If an obstetrician is not well trained, and he/she has practiced in an environment with poor quality control, the consequences can be enormous for both the mother and the baby.

In the summer of 2008, the Perinatal Unit at University of Tennessee Health Science Center (UTHSC) in Memphis started a reorganization of the perinatal program at Regional One Health (ROH). Our new program was designed to improve obstetrical and neonatal care. It included three overlapping phases: Observation, Awareness, and Implementation. The Observation phase examined the obstetrical and neonatal care provided at ROH, particularly, seeking opportunities for improvement.

We realized that different definitions were used for the same clinical conditions. For example, a survey on the definition of *tachysystole* among 42 doctors and nurses resulted in 12 different definitions. There was poor communication between obstetricians and neonatologists. There was no peer review of cases that ended with low cord pH, low Apgar scores, or other complications.

The Awareness phase consisted of meetings, discussions, and surveys, which included all personnel involved with the Department of Obstetrics and Gynecology, the Division of Neonatology, and the hospital administration.

The two phases above informed the Implementation phase. The simulation program became part of this phase. For a while, simulation was not well accepted in our department because it appeared "ridiculous" and challenging to the older obstetricians. Participating in a simulation scenario was uncomfortable for some faculty and nurses at the beginning. However, with time, the team was built, and the benefit of simulation was understood and appreciated.

Following our initial experience, a team of doctors and nurses traveled to other hospitals to learn what teams in diverse areas of the world had accomplished with their simulation programs.

Our program grew, and we started training other doctors at UTHSC annual academic meetings. When we decided to give a name to our program, we contemplated different options, but eventually we settled for the acronym Ob FAST (Feasible Approach to Simulation Training in Obstetrics). The enhanced patient safety improved our outcomes: the neonatal mortality for very low birth weight infants in our hospital was 20% *above* the expected value before the start of our program. It improved to 20% *below* expected a few years following the inception of our program.

Simulation is now part of our daily practice and we started exporting our experience. Visiting professors and research fellows who came to our institution became interested in our program. One of those visiting professors, Professor Xenia Li, took a keen interest. She practices in Zhengzhou University in Henan province, China; through our joint efforts, we were invited to start the Ob FAST program there. In April 2017, we traveled to Zhengzhou University where we trained doctors from 36 hospitals located throughout the Henan province that has a population of 150 million. Since then, they have started their own simulation program with two training Ob FAST courses every year. Professor Li and her team have trained three-hundred-fifty doctors (trainers) from different hospitals up to now. We were again invited to China in March 2019 to participate in the Ob FAST simulation training that was presented at a national level at the Chinese Society of Obstetrics and Gynecology meeting.

Acknowledgments

This book was initially designed for our trainees. However, due to the paramount role that simulation will play in obstetrics and after gaining more experience with the program, I decided to extend the number of simulation scenarios and to develop a guide that could be useful to all centers who would like to learn and start a simulation program. Most of the leaders involved in obstetric simulation at UTHSC in Memphis have collaborated with me in the development of this book. Dr. Danielle Tate, Dr. Ravpreet Gill, Karen Hamilton, and Bonnie Miller have played a paramount role in the training of nurses and doctors at UTHSC and at our annual meeting in Destin, Florida. Danielle, Bonnie, and Rav traveled with me to China to start the program there. Two of my clinical fellows, Dr. Pedro Argoti and Dr. Jennifer Barr, have spent long hours on this project and have collaborated with me in the organization and completion of this guide in a timely fashion, and Ms. Rosa Elvira Lucero and Dr. Francesco Napoleone have contributed to the completion of the project with their work on the iconography. Dr. Ravpreet Gill has contributed to the chapters on anesthesia, respiratory distress, and cardiac arrest in pregnancy. Ms. Karen Hamilton has contributed to the development of intrapartum fetal monitoring chapter. Ms. Bonnie Miller has participated in the completion of teamwork, intrapartum fetal monitoring, antepartum, and postpartum hemorrhage chapters. Dr. Danielle Tate has served as the director of the simulation program of the ob/gyn department, and she has contributed to the chapters on shoulder dystocia, vaginal breech, antepartum hemorrhage, and cord prolapse. Dr. Xenia Li has served as the director of the simulation program in China, and she has contributed to the uterine inversion chapter. Dr. Mauro Schenone, Ms. Jennifer Carelle, our sonographers, and Cameron Lowry have contributed to the ultrasound chapter. Dr. Sandeep Chilakala has contributed to the development of the neonatology simulation chapter. Dr. Molly Houser has contributed to the interstitial pregnancy section.

All ob nurses at Regional One Health have done a wonderful job over the years in collaborating with the doctors on developing and expanding our simulation program.

Last but not least, I thank Dr. Ken Brown, JD, MPA, PhD, FACHE, and his team for the state-of-the-art simulation center that they have created at UTHSC and for allowing us the use of some of the pictures of the center for this book.

About the Author

Dr. Giancarlo Mari was born in Salerno, Italy. Following the completion of his medical training and residency in obstetrics and gynecology at Napoli and Parma universities, he moved to the United States. In the United States, he obtained his MD, completed a residency in obstetrics and gynecology and a maternal fetal medicine fellowship at Yale University. He was at Yale for 10 years. Three years following the completion of his fellowship, he was promoted to associate professor at Yale.

Following other academic experiences as director of prenatal diagnosis, director of fetal therapy, director of maternal fetal medicine fellowship, and director of maternal fetal medicine, he became chairman of obstetrics and gynecology at the University of Tennessee Health Science Center in Memphis in 2009.

Dr. Mari's contribution to research and clinical practice include diagnosis and management of fetal anemia, Doppler ultrasonography, intrauterine growth restriction, twin-twin-transfusion syndrome, fetal therapy, infant mortality, and simulation in obstetrics.

Contents

CHAPTER 1

Teamwork Training: Basic Concepts

LEARNING OBJECTIVES

- Recognize the difference between technical and non-technical skills training.
- Describe the importance of teamwork training.
- List strategies for team-based safety training.

The goal of each obstetrician and each labor and delivery unit is a safe birth for both newborn and mother. In 2010, the Joint Commission published a Sentinel Event Alert about rising maternal mortality rates and our need to address them.[1] Up to half of the maternal deaths are preventable.[2] In 2001, the Institute of Medicine stated, "Health care organizations should establish interdisciplinary team training programs for clinicians to incorporate the proven team training strategies used in the aviation industry."[3] Since the publication of that report, a series of measures have been proposed and adopted in obstetrics and in medicine in general. Simulation training plays a paramount role in obstetrics for improving perinatal outcome.[2,4,5]

Management of any obstetric emergency requires both technical and non-technical skills. Technical skills include identifying the correct procedure and knowing how to do it. Examples are one's knowing the appropriate dose of epinephrine to give to a patient in anaphylaxis or knowing how to correctly apply forceps blades.

Non-technical skills can be more challenging to define but are essential to the success of an obstetrics team. These skills include communication with patients, partners, and team members, situational awareness, task management, and teamwork protocols.[2] Team members will benefit from practicing specific communication strategies, including the following (Fig. 1.1)[2,6]:

- **Call-out**—Clearly informing all team members regarding important information. For example, stating directly, "There is a cord prolapse."
- **Directed communication**—Using eye contact and names when possible. For example, "Sally, please start an IV."

- **Closed-loop communication**—Repeating back the information as communicated to ensure that it was properly received. For example, "Okay. I am starting an IV."

Both technical and non-technical skills can be developed through simulation. Simulation is used to avoid exposing patients to students' learning curves and to prepare health professionals to manage conditions that are not frequently experienced, but need to be managed promptly and effectively.[7] The practice of simulation in obstetrics in the United States was common in the 19th century when women delivered at home and not at the hospital.[8] With more deliveries occurring in hospitals, trainees were exposed to a large obstetric population and the simulation practice became unimportant. It has been rediscovered in the last 20 years.

Simulation can be adapted to fit the needs and budget of any department. It can be as simple as walking through the algorithm for treatment of antepartum hypertension or as complex as performing procedures on a high-fidelity mannequin. Simulations should be as realistic as possible with the materials available. Fig. 1.2 shows the plan of the simulation laboratory at the University of Tennessee Health Science Center (UTHSC) in Memphis. It is a state-of-the-art lab.

In 2008, we started a program that had as its goal the decrease of neonatal and infant mortality in our hospital. Simulation in obstetrics was part of this program. In a few years following the beginning of our program, the neonatal mortality for very low birth weight infants in our hospital decreased from 20% above the expected to 20% below the expected (Fig. 1.3) (Vermont Oxford Network).[9,10] All UTHSC faculty, students, fellows, and staff that rotate on labor and delivery undergo this simulation training.

Safety Training for Obstetric Emergencies. https://doi.org/10.1016/B978-0-323-69672-2.00001-1

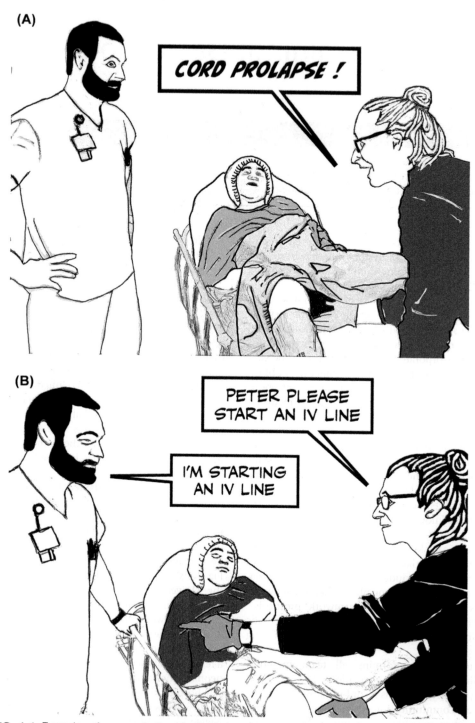

FIG. 1.1 Examples of communication strategies including call-out **(A)** and directed communication and closed-loop communication **(B)**.

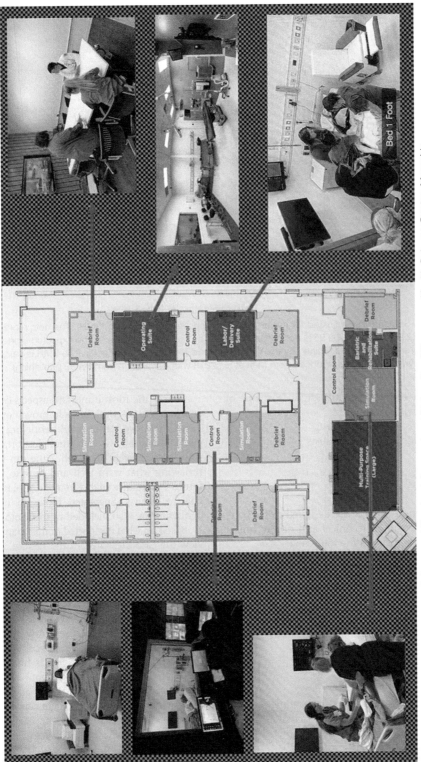

FIG. 1.2 Layout of the simulation center at University of Tennessee Health Science Center, Memphis.

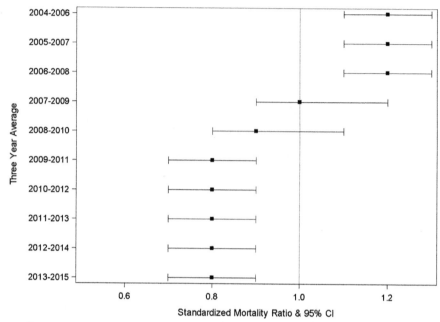

FIG. 1.3 Standard risk adjusted for mortality and composite morbidity ratio (SMR). The dots represent the mean; the bars represent the 95% confidence interval. The number 1 represents the expected mortality and composite morbidity as determined by the Vermont Oxford Network for our center. The SMR is calculated using a 3-year average (Reproduced from Mari et al., 2018 with permission from SAGE publishing)

The members of our team include at least one of each of the following disciplines:

- Anesthesiologists and anesthetists
- Maternal–fetal medicine specialists
- Midwifes
- Obstetricians
- Neonatologists
- Nurses

The chapters in this guide are designed to facilitate the development of both technical and non-technical skills. Each chapter includes the following:

1. Learning objectives
2. Material regarding the specific topic and required skills to manage a certain condition
3. References
4. Simulation
   a. Materials needed
   b. Key personnel
   c. Sample scenario
5. Simulation checklist
6. Debriefing

All of the above are important. The sample scenario can be used as a starting point for discussion and/or simulation. The checklist is usually completed by an observer for detailed evaluation of team performance during safety drills.

One of the most important aspects of teamwork is a commitment to continuous improvement in the future. To this end, we recommend debriefing as a team after every simulation and, even more importantly, after every real obstetric event. The debriefing can be as simple as reviewing what went well and how to improve in the future.[11] Certain scenarios may prompt more specific details to discuss. Suggested topics to include in your debriefing are also included in the sample scenarios.

Based on what is reported in this chapter, when we review the case presented in the Preface, many opportunities for the "team" become evident. There was no teamwork. There was a lack of technical and non-technical skills. With communication and good practice, perhaps the trauma to the patient, her baby, and to the families could have been avoided. Some observations and opportunities of that case follow: Why did the obstetrician admit his patient in one hospital where the doctors could not be trusted? It was his responsibility to follow his patient during the night—why had he failed in that responsibility? The patient had been fully dilated for less than one hour, and there was no fetal heart rate concern. Why was the vacuum applied?

The criticisms from the obstetrician to the team in front of the patient, in the delivery room and when the patient was being transferred, were not appropriate.

It is suggested that the obstetrician with his comments wanted to justify his negligence. The lack of a debrief, in this case is another primary concern. The second surgery did not appear to be justified, and not allowing the second opinion was a major breach. Starting antibiotics three days following the beginning of the fever was also not the best management when the patient was complaining of urinary burning.

There was a not-insignificant amount of arrogance in this case, "The arrogance of the ignorant." What would have been a normal, spontaneous delivery with joy for patient, the team, and her family became, as described by the patient and her family, a nightmare. This case emphasizes what Hippocrates said approximately 2500 years ago: Primum non nocere.

Training and simulation could have helped to decrease the sadness of such cases as the one presented here.

REFERENCES

1. Preventing maternal death. *Sentinel Event Alert*. 2010;(44): 1−4.
2. Morgan PJ, Tregunno D, Pittini R, et al. Determination of the psychometric properties of a behavioural marking system for obstetrical team training using high-fidelity simulation. *BMJ Qual Saf*. 2012;21(1):78−82.
3. Baker A. Crossing the quality chasm: a new health system for the 21st century. *BMJ*. 2001;323(7322):1192.
4. Draycott T, Sibanda T, Owen L, et al. Does training in obstetric emergencies improve neonatal outcome? *BJOG*. 2006;113(2):177−182.
5. Crofts J, Lenguerrand E, Bentham G, et al. Prevention of brachial plexus injury—12 years of shoulder dystocia training: an interrupted time-series study. *BJOG*. 2016; 123(1):111−118.
6. Kleinman ME, Goldberger ZD, Rea T, et al. 2017 American Heart Association focused update on adult basic life support and cardiopulmonary resuscitation quality: an update to the American Heart Association guidelines for cardiopulmonary resuscitation and emergency cardiovascular care. *Circulation*. 2018;137(1):e7−e13.
7. Owen H, Pelosi MA. A historical examination of the Budin-Pinard phantom: what can contemporary obstetrics education learn from simulators of the past? *Acad Med*. 2013;88(5):652−656.
8. Gardner R, Raemer DB. Simulation in Obstetrics and Gynecology. *Obstet Gynecol Clin N Am*. 2008;35:97−127.
9. Mari G, Bursac Z, Goedecke PJ, Dhanireddy R. Factors associated with improvements in mortality and morbidity rates of very-low-birth-weight infants: a cohort study. *Glob Pediatr Health*. 2018;5, 2333794X18765366.
10. Network VO. *What Is Vermont Oxford Network*; 2017. Available from: https://public.vtoxford.org/about-us/.
11. Corbett N, Hurko P, Vallee JT. Debriefing as a strategic tool for performance improvement. *J Obstet Gynecol Neonatal Nurs*. 2012;41(4):572−579.

Technical Skills	Non-Technical Skills
Medication dosing	Communication with team members
Obstetric maneuvers	Situational awareness
Surgical technique	Task management
Management algorithms	Teamwork

Technical and non-technical skill sets.

CHAPTER 2

Checklists in Obstetrics

LEARNING OBJECTIVES

- Recognize in what types of situations checklists are appropriate.
- Describe characteristics of good checklists.

The practice of obstetrics and medicine in general are increasing in complexity. With complex tasks, the risks for human error also increase. To cope with this complexity, the field of medicine has embraced a strategy successfully implemented in the airline industry: the checklist (Fig. 2.1).[1]

The goal of a checklist is to reduce a complex task to its simpler components. This identifies which steps are critical and which tasks should be delegated to whom. When used correctly, they promote consistency in team performance.[2]

The Society for Maternal Fetal Medicine has listed six types of procedures in which checklists may be useful[2]:

- Procedures with many steps
- Procedures in which failure to validate critical information could result in serious harm
- Procedures in which omission of a step could result in serious harm
- Procedures performed in high-stress situations
- Procedures with recently added new steps
- Procedures performed infrequently by a team

Effective checklists should be developed with input from all key members of the team. Each person can offer his/her own perspective on which tasks he/she is responsible. After its initial development, the checklists should be trialed in a simulation. Teams can then debrief and adapt the checklist before implementing it in a true clinical emergency.

Throughout this guide, we have included examples of checklists for the included clinical scenarios. They can be used when performing simulation drills and be adapted for implementation in clinical practice.

Obstetric teams will also benefit from implementing obstetric safety bundles that provide resources for an interdisciplinary team. Implementation of these

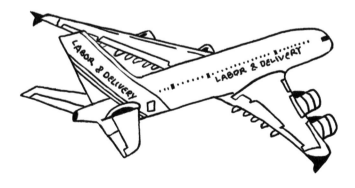
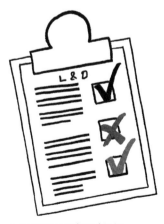

FIG. 2.1 Taking its cue from the airline industry, the field of obstetrics has now seen improved safety due to the implementation of checklists.

Safety Training for Obstetric Emergencies. https://doi.org/10.1016/B978-0-323-69672-2.00002-3

bundles assures that everyone in a facility works together to recognize and respond to mothers with potentially life-threatening conditions.[3] The California Maternal Quality Care Collaborative adapted this approach and has demonstrated a decrease in maternal mortality in California despite rising mortality nation-wide.[4] Readers will be able to find useful tools for implementing patient safety bundles on the Internet.[5,6]

REFERENCES

1. Clay-Williams R, Colligan L. Back to basics: checklists in aviation and healthcare. *BMJ Qual Saf.* 2015;24(7):428–431.

2. Bernstein PS, et al. The development and implementation of checklists in obstetrics. *Am J Obstet Gynecol.* 2017; 217(2):B2–B6.

3. Bernstein PS, et al. National Partnership for Maternal Safety: consensus bundle on severe hypertension during pregnancy and the postpartum period. *Obstet Gynecol.* 2017;130(2): 347–357.

4. Addressing maternal mortality and morbidity in California through public-private partnerships. *Health Aff.* 2018;37(9): 1484–1493.

5. Care CoPSiWsH. *Patient Safety Bundles;* 2018. Available from: https://www.cmqcc.org/resources-toolkits.

6. Collaborative CMQC. *Resources & Toolkits;* 2018. Available from: https://www.cmqcc.org/resources-toolkits.

Delivery Room Management of a Preterm Infant

Preterm delivery is defined as delivery at <37 weeks gestation. In United States, the preterm birth rate is 9.9% of all births[1]. With a history of preterm birth, there is a 22% increased risk of having a preterm birth in following pregnancy.[2] There is an inverse relationship between gestational age at delivery and the risk of neonatal morbidity and mortality.[3] Neonatal resuscitation is the most commonly provided form of resuscitation in the hospitals.[4] Approximately 6–10% of very low birthweight and extremely low birthweight infants are reported to receive extensive cardiopulmonary resuscitation at birth.[5] Teams providing neonatal resuscitation must always be prepared to provide this life-saving resuscitation at every delivery. Simulation-based training of the resuscitation teams will improve the cognitive, technical, and behavioral skills.[6] Newborn resuscitation training should be recurrent and should occur more frequently than once per year to maintain optimal performance.[7]

RISK FACTORS FOR PRETERM BIRTH

- African-American race
- Extremes of maternal age
- Multifetal gestation
- Preterm labor/preterm premature rupture of membranes
- Preeclampsia/eclampsia
- Fetal growth restriction
- Fetal anomalies
- Maternal substance abuse
- Uterine anomalies
- Placental abnormalities/abruptio placenta
- Trauma

DELIVERY ROOM CHECKLIST

General

- Room temperature 74–77°F
- Team briefing
  - Introduce and assign roles
  - *Ask the following four prebirth questions:*
    - What is the expected gestational age?
    - Is the amniotic fluid clear?
    - How many babies are expected?
    - Are there any additional risk factors?
- Assemble the necessary equipment and supplies

Nursing

- Radiant warmer on MANUAL and preheat, temperature probe and cover, hat, warm towels
- Bulb syringe
- Stethoscope
- Warming mattress, Neowrap or plastic bag if <32 weeks
- EKG leads
- Fluids/syringes and medications (normal saline, epinephrine 1: 10,000)
- Supplies for umbilical venous lines

Safety Training for Obstetric Emergencies. https://doi.org/10.1016/B978-0-323-69672-2.00003-5

- Supplies to document the events
- Know when and how to call for additional help if required

Respiratory therapy

- Surfactant and tubing
- Set up T piece resuscitator (initial settings PIP 20–25 cm H_2O, PEEP 5–6 cm H_2O (titrate PIP up, as needed) (Fig. 3.1)
- Flow-inflating or self-inflating bag (Fig. 3.2)
- Neonatal facemasks
- Laryngoscopes (straight blades with sizes 00,0 and 1) and endotracheal tubes (sizes 2.5, 3.0, 3.5) and LMA (size 1) (Fig. 3.3)
- Carbon dioxide detector
- Meconium aspirator
- Endotracheal tube securing device
- Oxygen (blender set to 21% (21%–30% if <35 weeks gestation))
- Pulse oximeter with sensor and cover
- Preductal target oxygen saturation card
- 10 or 12F suction catheter attached to wall suction, set at 80–100 mmHg

MANAGEMENT OF A PRETERM INFANT AT BIRTH PER NRP GUIDELINES
Preparing for the preterm birth

- Assemble the team
- Team briefing
- Assess perinatal risk factors
- Review roles and delegate tasks
- Review the checklist and perform equipment check

After delivery of the infant

- Assess the need for delayed cord clamping (per unit policy)
- Place the infant on the back under radiant warmer on warm blankets covered thermal mattress

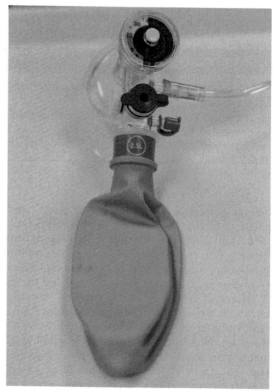

FIG. 3.2 Flow-inflating bag.

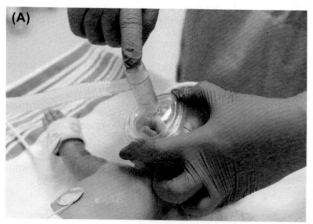

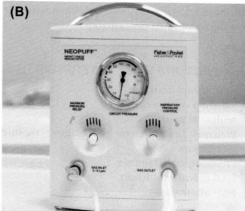

FIG. 3.1 Resuscitation with **(A)** T-piece adaptor and **(B)** Neopuff.

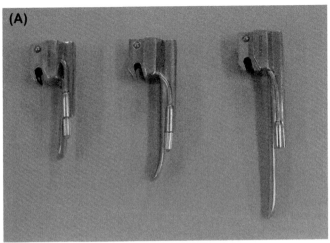 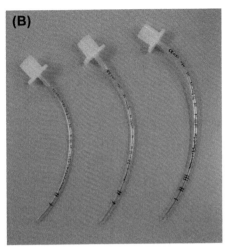

FIG. 3.3 Examples of **(A)** laryngoscopes and **(B)** endotracheal tubes.

- Position the head and neck in "sniffing" position
- Cover with plastic wrap
- Place a hat
- Assess breathing, heart rate (HR) with stethoscope and tone
- Stimulate. Suction gently only if necessary (mouth before nose)
- Place the temperature probe and change to servo-control
- Pulse oximeter probe to the right hand

Interventions based on assessment (Table 3.1)

TABLE 3.1	
Apnea OR Gasping Respirations OR Heart Rate <100 bpm	**Heart Rate >100 bpm and Labored Breathing**
Initiate positive pressure ventilation (PPV) (40−60 times per minute)	Trial of continuous positive airway pressure and observe for spontaneous respirations

Continued resuscitation

- Assess for clinical improvement (HR improving and chest rising) after 15 s of PPV
- Ventilation corrective steps "MR. SOPA" if no clinical improvement.

- Mask adjustment
- Reposition head
- Suction airway
- Open mouth
- Pressure increase
- Alternate airway
- Reassess after 30 s of PPV
- If clinical improvement, then continue PPV and gradually reduce the rate and monitor for spontaneous breathing
- If HR < 60 bpm, initiate chest compressions (Intubate if not already done)
- Call for additional help
- Increase the FiO_2 to 100%
- Coordinated chest compressions and ventilations (3 compressions + 1 breath every 2 s)
- Prepare and insert umbilical venous lines
- Assess the HR after 60 s
- If HR < 60 bpm, check the quality of compressions/ventilations and consider epinephrine (1: 10,000) intravenous (0.1−0.3 mL/kg) or endotracheal (0.5−1 mL/kg)
- Assess the HR 1 min after epinephrine administration
- Repeat the dose every 3−5 min if no improvement in the HR

Communication

- Effective communication between the team members
- Post-resuscitation team debriefing

Disposition

- Transfer to the neonatal intensive care unit

Documentation

- Documentation of the timeline of events

REFERENCES

1. Martin JA, Hamilton BE, Osterman MJK, Driscoll AK, Drake P. Births: Final data for 2017. *Natl Vital Stat Rep.* 2018;67(8):1–50.
2. Mercer BM, Goldenberg RL, Moawad AH, et al. The preterm prediction study: effect of gestational age and cause of preterm birth on subsequent obstetric outcome. National Institute of Child Health and Human Development Maternal-Fetal Medicine Units Network. *Am J Obstet Gynecol.* 1999;181(5 Pt 1):1216–1221.
3. Stoll BJ, Hansen NI, Bell EF, et al. Neonatal outcomes of extremely preterm infants from the NICHD Neonatal Research Network. *Pediatrics.* 2010;126(3):443–456.
4. Finer N, Rich W. Neonatal resuscitation for the preterm infant: evidence versus practice. *J Perinatol.* 2010;30(suppl):S57–S66.
5. Roehr CC, Hansmann G, Hoehn T, Buhrer C. The 2010 Guidelines on Neonatal Resuscitation (AHA, ERC, ILCOR): similarities and differences–what progress has been made since 2005? *Klin Pädiatr.* 2011;223(5):299–307.
6. Cheng A, Lang TR, Starr SR, Pusic M, Cook DA. Technology-enhanced simulation and pediatric education: a meta-analysis. *Pediatrics.* 2014;133(5):e1313–e1323.
7. Wyllie J, Perlman JM, Kattwinkel J, et al. Part 7: neonatal resuscitation: 2015 international consensus on cardiopulmonary resuscitation and emergency cardiovascular care science with treatment recommendations. *Resuscitation.* 2015;95:e169–201.

FURTHER READING

1. Weiner GM, ed. *Textbook of Neonatal Resuscitation.* 7th ed. Elk Grove Village (IL): American Academy of Pediatrics and American Heart Association; 2016.

Neonatal Resuscitation Simulation

MATERIALS NEEDED
- Manikin
- Neonatal resuscitation equipment

KEY PERSONNEL
- Neonatologist
- Neonatal nurse
- Respiratory therapist

SAMPLE SCENARIO
You are called to attend a delivery of a 25 weeks gestation preterm male infant being delivered via cesarean. Mother is an 18-year-old G1 P0 with preeclampsia with severe features. She received two doses of betamethasone. Mother's blood type is A+ and all other prenatal labs are within normal limits. No other significant past medical or surgical history. Fetal heart tracing showed nonreassuring fetal heart tracing pattern.

DEBRIEFING AND DOCUMENTATION
- Review the clinical events
- Participants' roles and their feelings
- Discuss the behavioral skills relevant to the scenario
- Importance of avoiding hypothermia
- Indications of PPV
- Effective PPV and MR. SOPA
- Indications of endotracheal intubation and chest compressions
- Need for additional help
- Umbilical venous lines
- Indications of epinephrine and need for volume resuscitation
- Communication with parents and family of the infant
- Disposition of the infant

Simulation Checklist		Time	Comments
Initial response	Assembled the team		
	Reviewed notes and delegated tasks		
	Assessed perinatal risk factors		
	Checked list and equipment		
Assessment of neonate	Placed infant under radiant warmer and on warm blankets covered thermal mattress		
	Sniffing position		
	Stimulated infant		
	Covered with plastic wrap		
	Placed hat		
	Assessed heart rate, breathing, tone		
	Pulse oximeter probe on right hand		
Apnea OR gasping OR HR < 100 bpm	Administered PPV using T- piece resuscitator		
	Starting FiO_2—30%		
	Assessed effectiveness of PPV		
	Assessed need for intubation		
	Initiated chest compressions if the HR < 60 bpm		
	Increased FiO_2 to 100% when chest compressions started		
	Coordinated chest compressions and ventilations		
	Assessed the HR after 60 s of chest compressions		
	Considered epinephrine		
Communication	Updated parents		
	Discussed need for additional help		
	Debriefed with team members		
Documentation	Timeline of events		
	Disposition of infant		

Technical Skills	Non-Technical Skills
Assemble resuscitative equipment	Communication with team members
Perform neonatal intubation	Assign team roles
Perform chest compressions	Task management
Describe neonatal resuscitation algorithms	Documentation

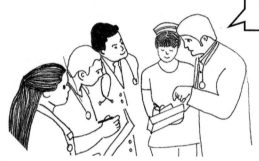

Technical and nontechnical skills for neonatal resuscitation.

CHAPTER 4

Cardiac Arrest in Pregnancy

LEARNING OBJECTIVES

- Describe principles of Basic Life Support.
- Describe principles of Advanced Cardiovascular Life Support as they relate to pregnancy.

The goal of this chapter is to highlight pregnancy-related pearls with regards to maternal resuscitation. This section presupposes knowledge of Basic Life Support and Advanced Cardiovascular Life Support (ACLS) training. Please see your local training agency if you require formal training Fig. 4.1 shows the basic equipment needed for cardiopulmonary. The most important thing to remember is the "ABCs"—airway, breathing, and circulation as summarized in Fig. 4.2.

BASIC LIFE SUPPORT[1]
Effective Chest Compressions (Fig. 4.3)

- Rate is 100−120 compressions per minute
- Compress the chest 5−6 cm (2−2.5 inches) with each downstroke
- Allow the chest to recoil completely after each downstroke
- To check adequacy → have another provider feel for femoral pulse during compressions
- Change the person doing compressions every 2−3 minutes to avoid fatigue

Ventilation

- Appropriate compression to ventilation ratio during CPR is 30 compressions to 2 breaths
- If an advanced airway is in place, give ventilations at a rate of approximately 10 per minute
- Ventilation rate can later be titrated based on blood gas values

Defibrillation (Fig. 4.4)

- Early defibrillation in patients with ventricular fibrillation improves outcomes
- Using the energy levels suggested by the manufacturer of the device—generally 360 J for a monophasic defibrillator and 200 J for a biphasic defibrillator

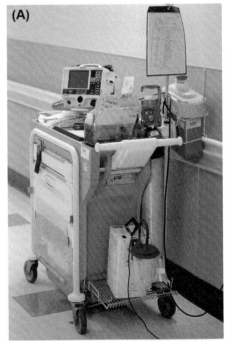

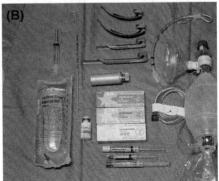

FIG. 4.1 Equipment for cardiopulmonary resuscitation including **(A)** code cart and **(B)** medications and respiratory equipment.

Safety Training for Obstetric Emergencies. https://doi.org/10.1016/B978-0-323-69672-2.00004-7

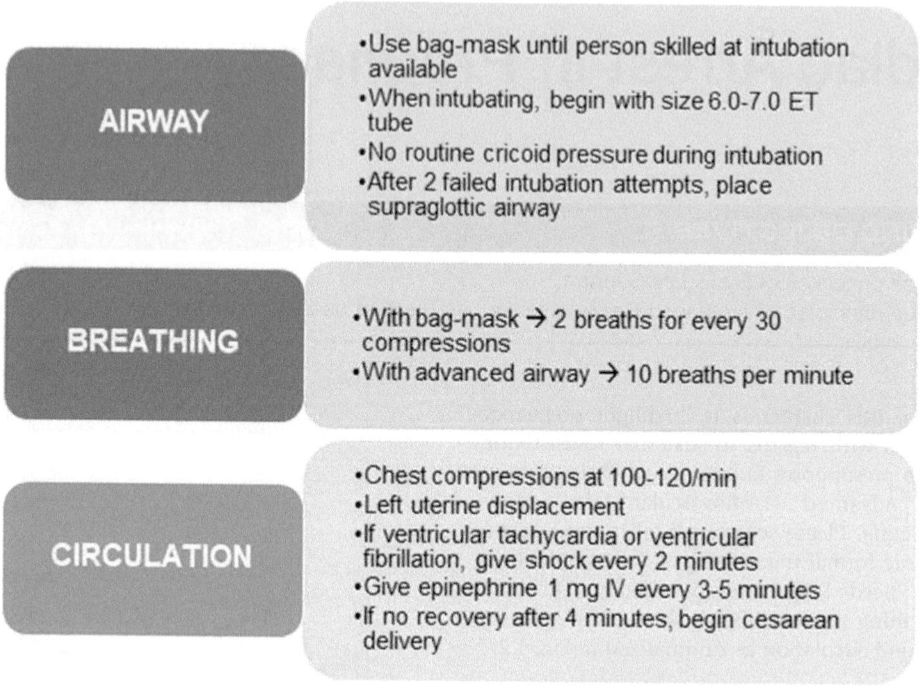

AIRWAY

- Use bag-mask until person skilled at intubation available
- When intubating, begin with size 6.0-7.0 ET tube
- No routine cricoid pressure during intubation
- After 2 failed intubation attempts, place supraglottic airway

BREATHING

- With bag-mask → 2 breaths for every 30 compressions
- With advanced airway → 10 breaths per minute

CIRCULATION

- Chest compressions at 100-120/min
- Left uterine displacement
- If ventricular tachycardia or ventricular fibrillation, give shock every 2 minutes
- Give epinephrine 1 mg IV every 3-5 minutes
- If no recovery after 4 minutes, begin cesarean delivery

FIG. 4.2 Essentials of cardiopulmonary resuscitation.

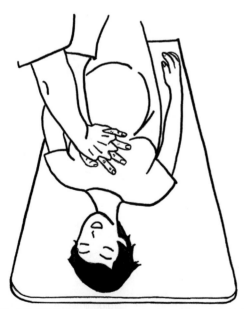

FIG. 4.3 Proper technique for chest compression. Hands should be placed on the lower half of the sternum. Each compression should have a depth of 5–6 cm with full recoil between compressions.

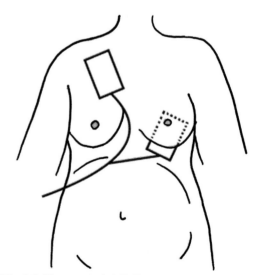

FIG. 4.4 Placement of defibrillator pads on right shoulder and left chest. The lateral pad should be placed under the patient's breast tissue.

- Resume CPR immediately after defibrillation—do not stop to check for pulse

ADVANCED CARDIOVASCULAR LIFE SUPPORT

General Pearls of Wisdom

- If you are giving any antiarrhythmic via a peripheral IV as opposed to a central line, raise the patient's arm and flush with 20 mL of saline

TABLE 4.1
Causes of Cardiac Arrest.

Hypovolemia	Toxins
Hypoxia	Tamponade (cardiac)
Hydrogen ion (acidosis)	Tension pneumothorax
Hypoglycemia	Thrombosis
Hypothermia	Trauma

- Try to identify and treat the underlying cause of the cardiac arrest using the classic mnemonic of the H's and T's (Table 4.1)
- Table 4.2 shows commonly needed medications

Considerations for ACLS in Pregnant Patients[2–5]

- IV access should be established *above the diaphragm*
- Left uterine displacement improves venous return (Fig. 4.5)
- When indicated, defibrillation should be performed in the usual manner
- Delivery of the fetus is part of resuscitation—the goal for delivery is within 5 minutes of the arrest. Perform C-section at bedside. Do not delay by taking patient to OR
- If a patient is receiving magnesium sulfate → stop it and give calcium chloride or calcium gluconate (1 g IV)
- Consider need for smaller (size 6.0–7.0) endotracheal tube in patients with airway edema
- After two failed intubation attempts, place a supraglottic airway
- Consider a pregnancy-specific differential for cardiac arrest[3] (Table 4.3)

TABLE 4.2
Medications Used in Maternal Resuscitation.

Medication	Dose	Indications
Epinephrine	1 mg IV every 3–5 minutes	Cardiac arrest (any rhythm)
Amiodarone	300 mg IV followed by 150 mg in 3–5 minutes	Shock-resistant ventricular fibrillation
Magnesium sulfate	2 g IV over 5–20 minutes	Torsades de pointes
Naloxone	2 mg intranasally or 0.4 mg IM/IV every 4 minutes	Opioid overdose with respiratory arrest
Atropine	0.5 mg IV every 3–5 minutes up to six doses	Bradycardia with poor perfusion
Sodium bicarbonate	1 mEq/kg	pH < 7.15 or prolonged arrest time

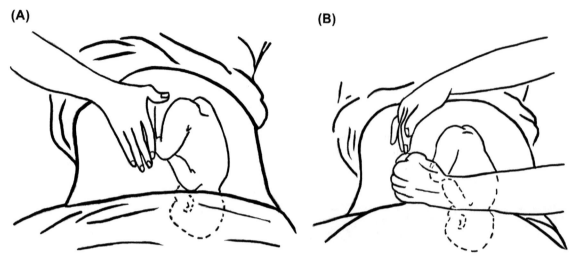

(A)   **(B)**

FIG. 4.5 Left uterine displacement using **(A)** 1-handed or **(B)** 2-handed technique.

TABLE 4.3
Causes of Cardiac Arrest in Pregnancy.
Anesthetic complications
Accidents/trauma
Bleeding
Cardiovascular
Drugs
Embolic disease
Fever/sepsis
General—the "H's and T's" listed earlier
Hypertension

REFERENCES

1. Kleinman ME, et al. 2017 American Heart Association focused update on Adult basic life support and cardiopulmonary resuscitation quality: an update to the American Heart Association guidelines for cardiopulmonary resuscitation and emergency cardiovascular care. *Circulation.* 2018; 137(1):e7—e13.
2. Lipman S, et al. The society for obstetric anesthesia and perinatology consensus statement on the management of cardiac arrest in pregnancy. *Anesth Analg.* 2014;118(5):1003—1016.
3. Jeejeebhoy FM, et al. Cardiac arrest in pregnancy: a scientific statement from the American Heart Association. *Circulation.* 2015;132(18):1747—1773.
4. Bennett TA, Katz VL, Zelop CM. Cardiac arrest and resuscitation unique to pregnancy. *Obstet Gynecol Clin N Am.* 2016; 43(4):809—819.
5. Zelop CM, et al. Cardiac arrest during pregnancy: ongoing clinical conundrum. *Am J Obstet Gynecol.* 2018;219(1):52—61.

Cardiac Arrest Simulation

MATERIALS NEEDED
- Manikin—should be able to at least perform chest compressions and intubation on manikin; a more realistic manikin will allow administration of medications and performance of an emergency cesarean delivery
- Laryngoscope
- Endotracheal tube
- Adult code cart—ideally participants would familiarize themselves with the defibrillator and the organization of the code cart available on your unit

KEY PERSONNEL
- Anesthesiologist
- Attending obstetrician
- Resident physician (if available in your institution)
- Two nurses

SAMPLE SCENARIO
A 24-year-old G1P0 female at 27 weeks gestation is brought to the Emergency Department after sustaining a motor vehicle accident. Just before you enter the room, she becomes unresponsive. There is no breathing or pulse noted. Her cardiac rhythm strip shows ventricular fibrillation.

DEBRIEFING AND DOCUMENTATION
- Time of arrest
- Time emergency cesarean delivery protocol initiated
- Time of infant delivery
- Time of return of spontaneous circulation
- Performance of left uterine displacement
- Detected rhythm
- Medications, shocks given
- Airway management
- Etiology of arrest
- Consideration of therapeutic hypothermia
- Communication with patient and family

Simulation Checklist		Time	Comments
Initial response	Apnea identified		
	Code called		
	Effective chest compressions initiated		
Team dynamics	Team leader identified		
	Team member roles clearly assigned		
Circulation	Correctly identified heart rhythm		
	Epinephrine 1 mg IV given		
	Subsequent medications given per ACLS protocol		
	Defibrillator called for		
	Correct strength on defibrillator used		
	Patient cart cleared before shock given		
Airway and breathing	100% oxygen attached to bag-mask ventilation		
	2-person bag-mask ventilation initiated		
	Effective bag-mask seal obtained		
	Pulse ox requested		
	Intubation tray requested		
	Intubation with 6.0–7.0 ET tube		
Pregnancy-related considerations	IV access obtained above diaphragm		
	Left uterine displacement		
	Fetal monitors removed		
	Decision made to proceed with cesarean		
	CPR continued during cesarean		
	Did not transport patient before cesarean		
	Delivery of infant within 5 minutes of arrest		
	Consideration given to causes of arrest		
Postresuscitation	Return of spontaneous circulation recognized		
	Considered therapeutic hypothermia		
Documentation	Persons present		
	Timing of medications		
	Timing of delivery		
	Timing of return of spontaneous circulation		
Communication	Call-out		
	Directed communication		
	Closed-loop communication		

Technical Skills	Non-Technical Skills
Demonstrate chest compression technique	Assign team roles
Demonstrate ventilation technique	Use closed-loop communication
Recognize shockable cardiac rhythms	Use directed communication
List dosages of ACLS medications	Task management

Let's debrief. . .

Technical and nontechnical skills for maternal resuscitation.

Respiratory Distress

SIGNS OF INCREASED WORK OF BREATHING

- Retractions and use of accessory muscles of respiration
- Inability to talk in full sentences
- Long pauses between sentences
- Orthopnea
- Sweating in a setting where it is not expected
- Restlessness, agitation, or decreased level of consciousness

WARNING SIGNS OF IMMINENT RESPIRATORY ARREST

- Decreased level of consciousness
- Paradoxical chest−abdomen movements
- Cyanosis

MANAGEMENT OF RESPIRATORY DISTRESS

Check for Airway Patency

- Look at the patient
- Listen over the neck and chest for abnormal sounds (Table. 5.1)

TABLE. 5.1
ABNORMAL AIRWAY SOUNDS AND WHAT THEY MEAN:
Snoring → obstruction of the airway
Inspiratory stridor → obstruction above the cords
Expiratory stridor → obstruction below the cords
Coarse lung sounds → secretions in the airway
Wheezing → flow restriction
Crackles → fluid or atelectasis at the alveolar level

Assess Work of Breathing

- For patients with increased work of breathing, assist ventilation according to Fig. 5.1.
- Tips for starting continuous positive airway pressure (CPAP):
  - Best with patient in a slightly sitting position
  - Requires good mask seal (Fig. 5.2).
  - Start with a pressure around 8−10 cm H_2O with an upper limit of around 20 cm H_2O
  - Be aware of increased risk of aspiration (Fig. 5.2)

Assess the Patient for Hypoxia ($SpO_2 \leq 94\%$)[1]

- Provide supplemental O_2 as needed
- FiO_2 increases 2%−3% for every L/minute flow

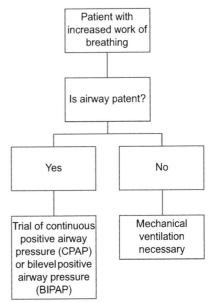

FIG. 5.1 Initial of a patient with increased work of breathing.

Safety Training for Obstetric Emergencies. https://doi.org/10.1016/B978-0-323-69672-2.00005-9

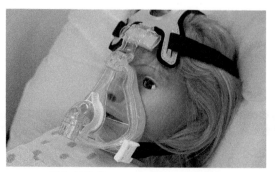

FIG. 5.2 Proper application of CPAP.

MANAGEMENT OF ANAPHYLAXIS[2]

- Remove any triggering agents
- Assess airway, breathing, and circulation
- Give **intramuscular epinephrine 0.5 mg of a 1:1000 (1 mg/mL)** solution
- If necessary, repeat epinephrine injection in 5–15 minutes
- Place patient in supine position with legs elevated
- Give supplemental oxygen as necessary

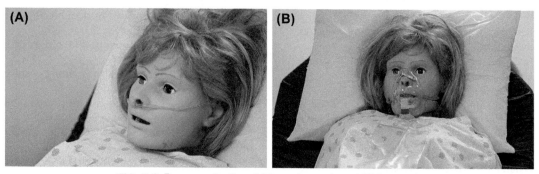

FIG. 5.3 Proper application of **(A)** nasal cannula and **(B)** facemask.

- Flow rates of different devices (Fig. 5.3):
  - Nasal cannula → 2–6 L/minute
  - Simple facemasks → 6–10 L/minute
  - Non-rebreather masks → 10–15 L/minute
- If the patient persistently needs a non-rebreather mask to maintain SpO_2 despite interventions, consider intubation

REFERENCES

1. Chestnut's Obstetric Anesthesia: Principles and Practice. p. 430–480.
2. Hernandez L, Papalia S, Pujalte GG. Anaphylaxis. *Primary Care.* 2016;43(3):477–485.

FURTHER READING

1. Zakowski M. Complications associated with regional anesthesia in the obstetric patient. *Semin Perinatol.* 2002;26(2): 154–168.
2. Balestrieri-Martinez B. Complications in obstetric anesthesia: nursing's role to anticipate, recognize, and respond. *J Perinat Neonatal Nurs.* 2009;23(1):23–30.
3. D'Angelo R, et al. Serious complications related to obstetric anesthesia: the serious complication repository project of the society for obstetric anesthesia and perinatology. *Anesthesiology.* 2014;120(6):1505–1512.

Respiratory Distress Simulation

MATERIALS NEEDED
- Manikin that will allow intubation
- Laryngoscope
- Endotracheal tube

KEY PERSONNEL
- Anesthesiologist
- Attending obstetrician
- Resident physician (if available in your institution)
- Nurse

SAMPLE SCENARIO
A 36-year-old G3P2002 female at 31 weeks gestation presents complaining of shortness of breath. She has a history of asthma but has not had her inhalers since her insurance lapsed 1 month ago. This evening, there was a house fire in her neighborhood that triggered her worsening symptoms. On presentation, her respiratory rate is 28 and her SpO_2 is 92%. She is unable to speak in complete sentences.

DEBRIEFING AND DOCUMENTATION
- Vital signs
- Assessment of airway
- Assessment of work of breathing
- Assessment of oxygenation
- Interventions
- Current maternal, fetal status
- Communication with patient and family

Simulation Checklist

		Time	Comments
Initial assessment	Checked for airway patency		
	Auscultated over neck and chest for abnormal sounds		
	Assessed work of breathing		
	Assessed hypoxia		
	Assessed peak flow rate		
	Initiated fetal monitoring		
Asthma interventions	Supplemental oxygen given and titrated for SpO_2 >95%		
	Albuterol nebulizer (2.5—5 mg) given		
	Inhaled ipratropium bromide given		
	Systemic steroids given		
	Consideration given to need for mechanical ventilation		
Documentation	Timing of medications		
	Response to medications		
Communication	Call-out		
	Directed communication		
	Closed-loop communication		
	Communication with patient		

Technical Skills	Non-Technical Skills
List signs of increased work of breathing	Recognize change in patient status
Recognize abnormal airway sounds	Communicate with team members
Initiate CPAP therapy	Task management
List indications for intubation	Teamwork

Technical and nontechnical skills for respiratory distress.

Anesthesia Complications

The most common modes of anesthesia used in obstetrics are neuraxial and general anesthesia. Examples of neuraxial anesthesia include epidural anesthesia and spinal anesthesia. This chapter begins with potential complications of neuraxial anesthesia. Fig. 6.1 demonstrates the important anatomy for these neuraxial anesthesia techniques. At the end of this chapter, we also discuss the complications of general anesthesia.

INTRAVASCULAR INFUSION OF LOCAL ANESTHETIC[1]

Pathophysiology

- Results from cannulation of blood vessels by the epidural catheter
- Usually prevented by giving a small "test dose" of lidocaine and epinephrine to test for intravascular placement or unrecognized placement in the spinal space *before* full dose is given

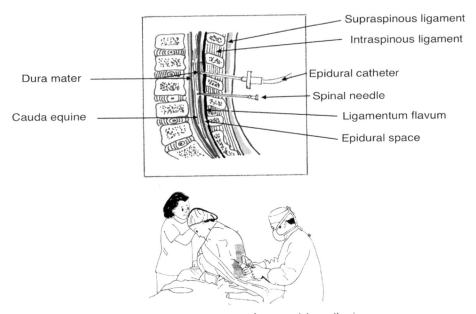

FIG. 6.1 Relevant anatomy for neuraxial anesthesia.

Safety Training for Obstetric Emergencies. https://doi.org/10.1016/B978-0-323-69672-2.00006-0

Symptoms

- "Ringing" or "buzzing" in the ears
- "Funny" or "metallic" taste in the mouth
- Tingling sensation around the lips
- Muscular twitching
- Loss of consciousness
- Cardiac arrest

Management

- Supportive care
- Stop epidural infusion
- Reassure patient that symptoms will resolve
- If appropriate and possible, replace the epidural catheter
- If the patient has bupivacaine-induced cardiac arrest, give Intralipid 20% bolus (1.5 mg/kg), followed by continuous intravenous infusion of 0.25 mg/kg for 60 minutes[2]

HIGH/TOTAL LEVEL OF SPINAL ANESTHESIA[3]

Risk Factors

- Unrecognized placement of the epidural catheter in the subarachnoid space
- Performance of a spinal following an inadequate epidural where an infusion was previously running via a catheter

Symptoms

- Dizziness
- Shortness of breath
- Weakness in hands
- Sudden agitation (may be due to hypoxia or relative hypotension)

Management

- Supportive care
- Patients may need their breathing assisted with a bag-valve mask
- Stop infusion of local anesthetic
- Assess the level of the block to either a difference in temperature (using alcohol or ice) or a difference in sharp touch, remembering these dermatomes (Fig. 6.2):
  - T4 = nipple line
  - T6 = xiphoid process
  - T10 = umbilicus
- Use level of block to monitor symptom progression/resolution

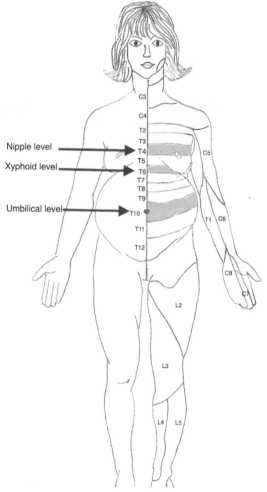

FIG. 6.2 Sensory assessment of dermatomes is used to determine level of neuraxial anesthesia.

HYPOTENSION

Pathophysiology

- Local anesthetic blockade of autonomic fibers results in vasodilation
- Vasodilation results in decreased cardiac preload and consequent hypotension

Management

- Manually displace the uterus or tilt the patient to one side (usually left lateral) to increase blood return to the heart (Fig. 6.3)
- Administer a fluid bolus (500 mL of normal saline)
- Administer vasopressors as needed (phenylephrine or ephedrine)

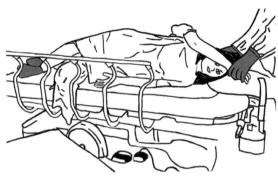

FIG. 6.3 Left lateral positioning reduces compression of inferior vena cava and improves blood flow to the uterus.

- If hemorrhage or severe anemia is considered to be a contributing factor, then consider blood products
- Assess the level of the block and consider stopping/decreasing the rate of the epidural infusion

POSTDURAL PUNCTURE HEADACHE[4,5]

Risk Factors
- Accidental puncture of the dura during placement of epidural catheter
- Deliberate puncture of the dura to provide spinal anesthesia

Symptoms
- Positional (minimal to no headache when supine and worse when sitting or standing)
- Onset typically 24−48 hours after puncture (but may be more delayed)
- May be frontal, occipital, or both

Management
- Usually resolves in 7 days, even without intervention
- Analgesics, especially oxycodone/acetaminophen and ketorolac
- Caffeine
- Oral sumatriptan
- Oral hydration
- Abdominal binder

TABLE 6.1
Agents That Can Trigger Malignant Hyperthermia
Halothane
Isoflurane
Sevoflurane
Desflurane
Enflurane
Succinylcholine

- Only definitive management is epidural blood patch
  - Both diagnostic and therapeutic
  - More likely to fail if performed less than 24 hours after dural puncture

MALIGNANT HYPERTHERMIA[6]

Pathophysiology
- Results from genetic disorder affecting calcium channel in skeletal muscle
- Exposure to certain anesthetic agents triggers uncontrolled calcium release (Table 6.1)
- Calcium triggers sustained muscle contraction and hypermetabolic state
- This triggers a cascade including skeletal muscle damage, hyperthermia, renal failure, and cardiac arrest

Signs and Symptoms
- Unexplained rise in end-tidal carbon dioxide
- Tachycardia
- Hyperthermia
- Arrhythmia
- Muscle rigidity

Management
- Stop triggering anesthetic agents
- Stop procedure as soon as possible
- Call Malignant Hyperthermia Hotline (1-800-644-9737)
- Hyperventilate with 100% oxygen at flows of 10 L/min
- If available, insert activated charcoal filters into breathing circuit

- Give dantrolene 2.5 mg/kg through large bore IV—repeat as needed until clinical response
- Obtain blood gas and serum sample to check for hyperkalemia
- Cool patient to below 38°C

REFERENCES

1. El-Boghdadly K, Chin KJ. Local anesthetic systemic toxicity: continuing professional development. *Can J Anaesth.* 2016; 63(3):330–349.
2. Whiteman DM, Kushins SI. Successful resuscitation with intralipid after marcaine overdose. *Aesthet Surg J.* 2014; 34(5):738–740.
3. Balestrieri-Martinez B. Complications in obstetric anesthesia: nursing's role to anticipate, recognize, and respond. *J Perinat Neonatal Nurs.* 2009;23(1):23–30.
4. Gaiser RR. Postdural puncture headache: an evidence-based approach. *Anesthesiol Clin.* 2017;35(1):157–167.
5. Katz D, Beilin Y. Review of the alternatives to epidural blood patch for treatment of postdural puncture headache in the parturient. *Anesth Analg.* 2017;124(4):1219–1228.
6. Hirshey Dirksen SJ, et al. Developing effective drills in preparation for a malignant hyperthermia crisis. *AORN J.* 2013; 97(3):329–353.

FURTHER READING

1. Zakowski M. Complications associated with regional anesthesia in the obstetric patient. *Semin Perinatol.* 2002;26(2): 154–168.
2. D'Angelo R, et al. Serious complications related to obstetric anesthesia: the serious complication repository project of the society for obstetric anesthesia and perinatology. *Anesthesiology.* 2014;120(6):1505–1512.

Anesthesia Complications Simulation

MATERIALS NEEDED
- Manikin or volunteer to act as patient

KEY PERSONNEL
- Anesthesiologist
- Attending obstetrician
- Resident physician (if available in your institution)
- Nurse

SAMPLE SCENARIO

A 26-year-old G2P1001 at 38 weeks gestation presents in active labor. She receives an epidural. A few minutes later, she complains to her nurse of ringing in her ears and a metallic taste in her mouth. As the nurse is speaking with her, the patient loses consciousness.

DEBRIEFING AND DOCUMENTATION
- Vital signs
- Medications infused through epidural
- Supportive measures initiated
- Disposition of epidural catheter
- Current maternal, fetal status
- Most likely diagnosis
- Communication with patient and family

Simulation Checklist

		Time	Comments
Initial response	Called for help		
	Recognized diagnosis of acute local anesthetic toxicity		
Airway	Checked airway		
	Inserted airway if necessary		
Breathing	Checked for spontaneous respirations		
	Supported respiration as necessary		
	Administered 100% oxygen		
Circulation	Checked for pulse		
	Considered need for cardiopulmonary bypass		
	Placed cardiac leads and assessed rhythm		
Other	Stopped epidural infusion		
	Considered use of medication to suppress seizure		
	Considered administration of 20% lipid emulsion		
Communication	Call-out		
	Directed communication		
	Closed-loop communication		
	Communication with patient		

Technical Skills	Non-Technical Skills
List signs and symptoms of anesthesia complications, including intravascular infusion of local anesthetic, high spinal level, hypotension, and postdural puncture headache	Communicate with patient and family about complications and interventions
List interventions for neuraxial anesthesia complications	Task management

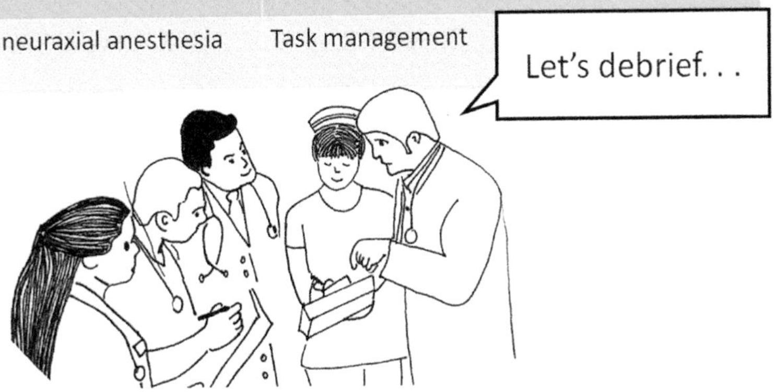

Let's debrief...

FIG. 6.4 Technical and nontechnical skills for anesthesia complications.

CHAPTER 7

Obstetric Ultrasound

IMAGE OPTIMIZATION

- Control deck, probe type, frequency, and orientation
  - The ultrasound control panel and keyboard share several common knobs and button even across brands. Such common controls include ultrasound modes, gain, depth, focal zone, and zoom (Fig. 7.1)
  - Most common probe used is a curvilinear array with a frequency 5 MHz for transabdominal approach. Transvaginal ultrasound can be used in selected situations
  - Please note the notch that indicates correct probe orientation (Fig. 7.2). Such notch should be maintained between 9 and 12 o'clock positions to avoid obtaining false laterality information (mirror image). If you are unable to ascertain laterality in an unfamiliar ultrasound machine, you can always press with a finger on each side of the probe and see in the screen which side of the screen such area is represented
  - Do not forget to apply ultrasound conductive gel!
- Ultrasound modalities
  - B-mode, also known as 2D, is the most used (Fig. 7.3)
  - M-mode detects movement of tissue, such as the cardiac ventricular walls. This modality allows for detection of fetal heart activity and to measure fetal heart rate. It is the preferred mode to

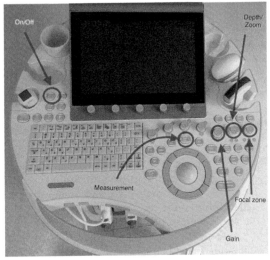

FIG. 7.1 Ultrasound control panel allows operator to adjust mode, gain, depth, and zoom.

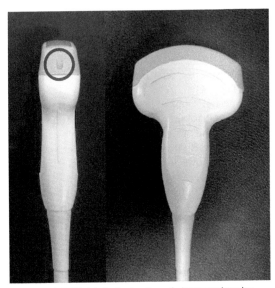

FIG. 7.2 Notch indicates top of ultrasound probe.

Safety Training for Obstetric Emergencies. https://doi.org/10.1016/B978-0-323-69672-2.00007-2

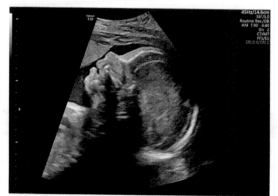

This image of a fetal profile is an example of B-mode ultrasound.

FIG. 7.3 B-mode presents with a 2D image of the area being studied.

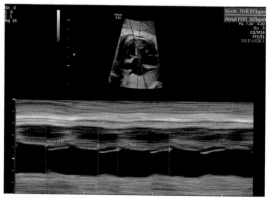

FIG. 7.4 M-mode detects movement of tissue, such as the cardiac ventricular walls. This modality allows for detection of fetal heart activity.

measure the fetal heart rate in early pregnancy (Fig. 7.4)
- Spectral Doppler is also used to assess blood flow. Place the sample gate in the four-chamber area and activate Spectral Doppler to obtain fetal heart rate blood flow Doppler waveforms. This allows for calculation of fetal heart rate (Fig. 7.5)
- Color Doppler: this modality produces color signals in the screen in areas of blood flow. In emergencies, it is also a useful tool to determine if the fetus is alive. When confirming no fetal heart activity, it may be helpful to open the color Doppler box (Fig. 7.6)

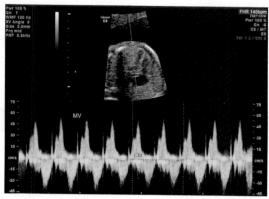

FIG. 7.5 Spectral Doppler is also used to assess blood flow. Place the sample gate in the four-chamber area and activate Spectral Doppler to obtain fetal heart rate blood flow Doppler waveforms.

- Ultrasound adjustment
  - Gain: Adjusting the gain will make the image brighter or darker. Too much or little gain will make things indistinguishable from each other in an either very bright or dark screen, respectively. Adjust the gain to reach a balance that allows you to better see the area of interest (Fig. 7.7)
  - Focal zone: Generally, the focal zone marker is best placed at the deepest level of the area of interest or slightly deeper (Fig. 7.8)
  - Depth: It allows the operator to adjust the depth of the area represented in the screen. Adjust the depth to exclude deep areas of no value and thus optimize visualization of the area of interest. In general, the area of interest should fill two thirds of the screen (Fig. 7.9)
  - Zoom: This tool magnifies the area of interest. It is recommended that the operator magnifies the area of interest to have it occupy two thirds of the screen (Fig. 7.10)

OBTAINING KEY ELEMENT OF OBSTETRIC ULTRASOUND DURING AN EMERGENCY
Pregnancy Location and Presentation

- It is a good habit to start your ultrasound examination from the uterine cervix and demonstrate the relationship of the cervix with presenting fetal part. This will confirm that the pregnancy is intrauterine and not an ectopic pregnancy. The bladder serves as a landmark that helps with orientation

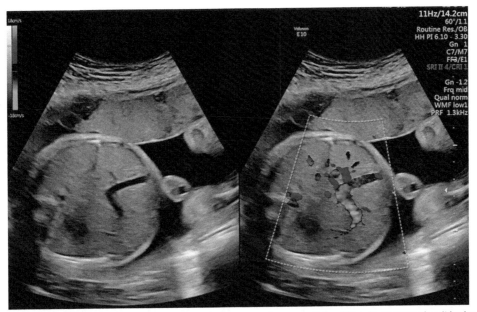

FIG. 7.6 Color Doppler produces color signals in the screen in areas of blood flow. In emergencies, it is also a useful tool to determine if the fetus is alive.

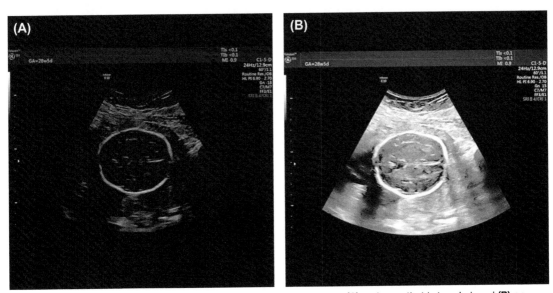

FIG. 7.7 Adjusting the gain will make the image brighter or darker: **(A)** an image that is too dark and **(B)** an image that is overcorrected.

- Starting to image from the cervix will also allow the examiner to determine the fetal presentation (the fetal part closest to the cervix, e.g., cephalic, breech, funic, complex). When none of these is present, consider transverse lie

Fetal Number

- Scanning the entire uterine cavity by sweeping the ultrasound probe side to side and cephalic to caudal is key to avoid missing a twin gestation. In addition,

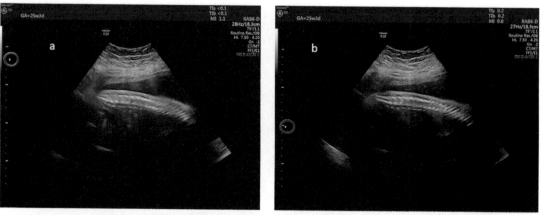

FIG. 7.8 The focal zone marker is best placed at the deepest level of the area of interest or slightly deeper. The interest intmis image is the fetal spine.

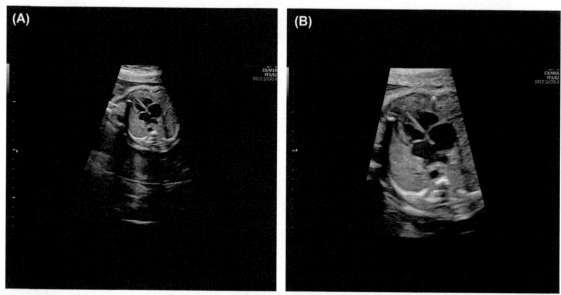

FIG. 7.9 Depth allows the operator to adjust the depth of the area represented in the screen. Adjust the depth to exclude deep areas of no value and thus optimize visualization of the area of interest: **(A)** the depth set is too deep and **(B)** improvement of the image with proper depth setting.

allow enough depth to cover the uterine cavity to the posterior wall

Fetal Heart Activity and Heart Rate

- B-mode generally suffices to detect fetal cardiac activity
- Color Doppler will show color signals in the cardiac area, if there is heart activity

- To determine fetal heart rate, M-mode (see Fig. 7.4) offers enough accuracy with less energy exposure than spectral Doppler (generally preferred to be compliant with ALARA principle especially in the first trimester). Spectral Doppler can also be used to measure the fetal heart rate (see Fig. 7.5). The ultrasound systems will usually display the option for measuring heart rate when freezing the image on M-mode or spectral

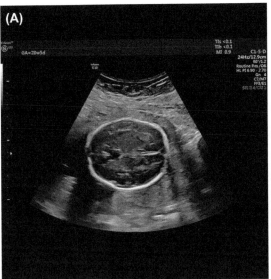 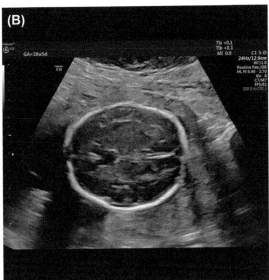

FIG. 7.10 Zoom magnifies the area of interest. It is recommended that the operator magnifies the area of interest to have it occupy two thirds of the screen: **(A)** an image with inadequate zoom and **(B)** improvement of the image with adjustment of zoom.

Doppler and/or activating the measurement menu (see Fig. 7.1). Place calipers at the same point of the cardiac cycle in two contiguous heart cycles
- When diagnosing a fetal demise, it is recommended to use more than one of these tools (e.g., B-mode, color Doppler, M-mode, or spectral Doppler)

Amniotic Fluid Volume

- When measuring amniotic fluid, the patient should be supine and the ultrasound probe should be held perpendicular to the long axis of the patient and perpendicular to the ground
- There are three ways of assessing amniotic fluid volume
  - Maximum vertical pocket: the deepest amniotic fluid pocket of all four quadrants (preferred method)
  - Amniotic fluid index (AFI): Used at 24 weeks of gestation or beyond. The maternal abdomen/uterus is divided into four imaginary quadrants. The deepest pocket of amniotic fluid in each quadrant is measured. The AFI is calculated by adding the deepest pocket of amniotic fluid for each of the four quadrants
  - Subjective assessment

Placental Location and Anatomy

- The placental echogenicity is usually unique and different from the adjacent myometrium, amniotic

fluid, or fetal parts. Becoming familiar with the placental shape and echogenicity is paramount to accurately assess placental location. Doppler color helps identifying the vascularity of the placental tissue
- In urgent or emergent situations, placental location may provide information to determine mode of delivery. In general, placenta previa is a contraindication for vaginal delivery and indicates a cesarean
- Ultrasound cannot completely rule out placental abruption but can be useful in identifying large retroplacental hematomas. When the abruption is large enough to be seen in ultrasound, the appearance will depend on the longevity of the abruption[1,2]
  - Acute hematoma appears generally hyperechoic or isoechoic to the placenta
  - Subacute hematoma may appear heterogeneous echogenicity or even hypoechoic (generally within 1 week)
  - Chronic hematoma appears sonolucent (2 weeks or more)

Fetal Biometry and Gestational Age

- Ultrasound plays a major role in determining the gestational age. The calculation is based on biometry variables such as femur length (FL), abdominal circumference (AC), head circumference (HC), and biparietal diameter (BPD)

- An accurate assessment of the gestational age is paramount when making decision about pregnancy and formulating a plan. Fetal viability is a key factor when making therapeutic decisions during

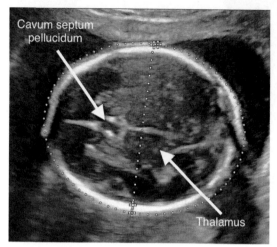

FIG. 7.11 The head circumference (HC) is measured on an image showing a transverse section of the fetal head. The following landmarks should be visualized: thalami (*open arrows*), cavum septum pellucidum (*solid arrow*), and midline falx (lines). The biparietal diameter is measured on the same image.

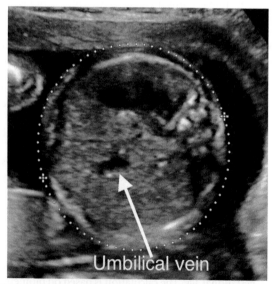

FIG. 7.12 Abdominal circumference (AC) is measured in a transverse section through the fetal abdomen at the level of the stomach and the intraabdominal portion of the umbilical vein–portal vein confluence.

pregnancy. Level of monitoring and intervention for fetal reasons depend on the level of viability. Dating by ultrasound is recommended when the discrepancy between ultrasound dating and last menstrual period is more than 5 days at less than 9 weeks, more than 7 days between 9 and 15 6/7 weeks, more than 10 days between 16 and 21 6/7 weeks, more than 14 days between 22 and 27 6/7 weeks, and more than 21 days at 28 weeks and beyond[3]

- The HC is measured on an image showing a transverse section of the fetal head. The following landmarks should be visualized: thalami and cavum septum pellucidum (Fig. 7.11)[4]
- The BPD should be measured on the same image as the HC described above. One caliper should be placed at the outer surface of the proximal parietal bone and the other caliper is placed on the inner

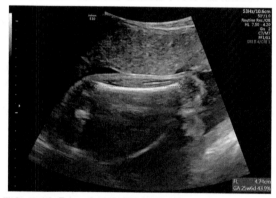

FIG. 7.13 Femur length (FL) is measured on a longitudinal image of the femur. The measured area should only include the diaphysis.

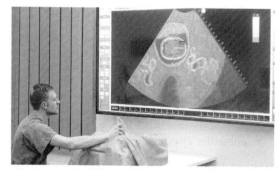

FIG. 7.14 Ultrasound simulator by Vimedix ultrasound simulator by CAE healthcare. This program simulator is used to train our medical students, residents, and faculty.

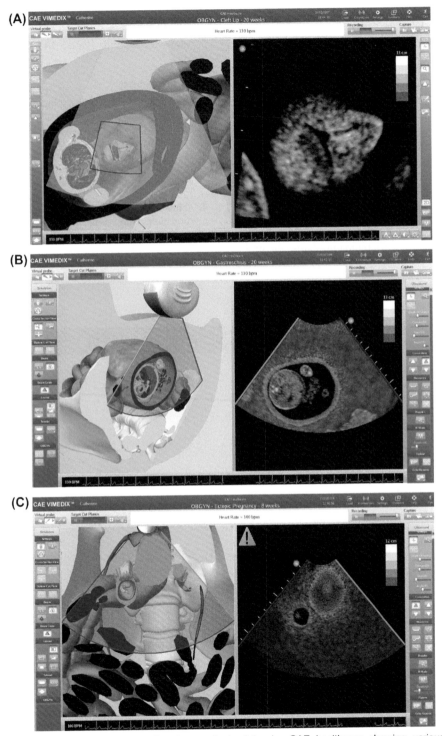

FIG. 7.15 Screenshots from Vimedix utrasound simulator by CAE healthcare showing various fetal pathology: **(A)** cleft lip, **(B)** gastroschisis, and **(C)** ectopic pregnancy.

surface of the distal parietal bone perpendicular to the midline falx (Fig. 7.11)[4]

- AC is measured in a transverse section through the fetal abdomen at the level of the intra-abdominal portion of the umbilical vein–portal vein confluence. Optimally, the full length of one rib should be visible on either side of the abdomen (Fig. 7.12)[4]
- FL is measured on a longitudinal image of the femur. The measured area should only include the diaphysis. The long axis of the femur should be perpendicular to the sound beam[4] (Fig. 7.13)

ULTRASOUND SIMULATION

- Use of an ultrasound simulator can allow the clinician to gain experience by manipulating the probe

- This allows the clinician to become facile with image acquisition without exposing patients to unnecessary ultrasounds (Figs. 7.14–7.15)

REFERENCES

1. Nyberg DA, et al. Sonographic spectrum of placental abruption. *AJR Am J Roentgenol.* 1987;148(1):161–164.
2. Woodward PJ. *Diagnostic Imaging. Obstetrics.* 2nd ed. Salt Lake City, Utah: Amirsys; 2011.
3. Committee on Obstetric Practice, t.A.I.o.U.i.M, M. the Society for Maternal-Fetal. Committee opinion No 700: methods for estimating the due date. *Obstet Gynecol.* 2017; 129(5):e150–e154.
4. Abuhamad A, et al. Obstetric and gynecologic ultrasound curriculum and competency assessment in residency training programs: consensus report. *Am J Obstet Gynecol.* 2018;218(1):29–67.

Ultrasound Simulation

MATERIALS NEEDED
- Standardized patient or ultrasound phantom
- Ultrasound machine
- Ultrasound gel

KEY PERSONNEL
- Attending obstetrician
- Resident physician (if available in your institution)

SAMPLE SCENARIO
A 25-year-old G1P0 at 32 weeks gestation presents with decreased fetal movement for the past 2 days. Demonstrate your ability to complete an ultrasound assessment of the fetus.

DEBRIEFING AND DOCUMENTATION
- Fetal number
- Fetal position
- Fetal cardiac activity
- Fetal movement
- Amniotic fluid assessment
- Placental location

Simulation Checklist		Time	Comments
Image optimization	Correct probe orientation		
	Gain		
	Depth		
	Focal zone		
	Zoom		
Documentation	Fetal number		
	Fetal position		
	Amniotic fluid assessment		
	Placental location		
Communication	Communication of findings with patient		
	Communication of findings with team		

Technical Skills	Non-Technical Skills
Determine pregnancy location and position	Communication with team members
Determine fetal number	Communication with patient
Assess fetal heart rate	Task management
Measure amniotic fluid volume	

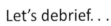

Let's debrief. . .

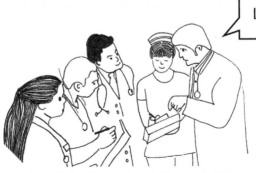

Technical and nontechnical ultrasound skills.

Intrapartum Fetal Monitoring

Fetal heart rate monitoring is the most common obstetric procedure, and yet it remains a frustrating technology, plagued by false-positive results and miscommunication between providers.

PHYSIOLOGIC BASIS FOR FETAL HEART RATE MONITORING

The goal of fetal heart rate monitoring is to assess fetal well-being.[1] A normal fetal heart rate tracing requires normal oxygenation of the mother and normal placental transfer of oxygen to the fetus. Any process that causes a break in the oxygen pathway can cause fetal heart rate abnormalities. Understanding this physiology is important to intervening to improve fetal oxygenation. Potential breaks in the oxygen pathway are summarized as follows:

- Maternal lungs
  - Respiratory depression (narcotics, magnesium)
  - Pneumonia/ARDS
  - Pulmonary embolus
  - Pulmonary edema
  - Asthma
  - Atelectasis
- Maternal heart
  - Reduced cardiac output
  - Hypovolemia
  - Decreased venous return (compression of vena cava)
- Maternal vasculature
  - Hypotension
  - Regional anesthesia
  - Medications (hydralazine, labetalol, nifedipine)
- Uterus
  - Excessive uterine activity
- Placenta
  - Placental abruption
- Umbilical cord
  - Cord compression
  - "True knot" in cord

FETAL HEART MONITORING COMPONENTS[2–4]

Baseline

- Defined as the average heart rate (rounded to the nearest five beats per minute) during a 10-minute segment
- Must be present for a minimum of 2 minutes within the 10-minute segment; if not, baseline is characterized as "indeterminant"
- Normal is 110–160 beats per minute

Variability

- Refers to the beat-to-beat changes in the baseline fetal heart rate (Fig. 8.1)
- Amplitude of variability is classified as follows:
  - Absent—no detectable variation
  - Minimal—detectable variation, but variation is five beats per minute or less
  - Moderate—6–25 beats per minute (this is normal)
  - Marked—greater than 25 beats per minute

Safety Training for Obstetric Emergencies. https://doi.org/10.1016/B978-0-323-69672-2.00008-4

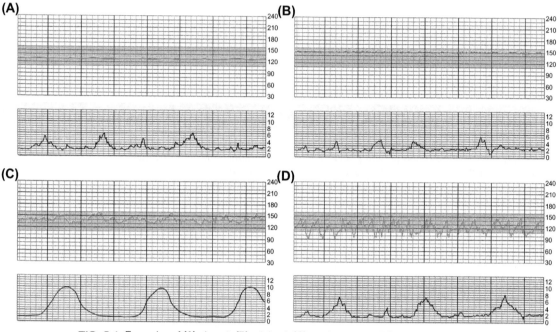

FIG. 8.1 Examples of **(A)** absent, **(B)** minimal, **(C)** moderate, and **(D)** marked variability.

Accelerations

- This is an abrupt rise in the fetal heart rate from the baseline
- Defined as follows:
  - At 32 weeks gestation or higher-peak of at least 15 beats per minute above the baseline and lasts at least 15 seconds
  - Prior to 32 weeks gestation-peak of at least 10 beats per minute above the baseline and lasts at least 10 seconds
  - At any gestation—a "prolonged acceleration" lasts 2−10 minutes
- Accelerations indicate that fetal acidemia is not present at that time

Decelerations (Fig. 8.2)

- Early decelerations
  - Onset to nadir of deceleration is 30 seconds or longer
  - Nadir of deceleration coincides with peak of contraction
- Late decelerations
  - Onset to nadir of deceleration is 30 seconds or longer

- Nadir of deceleration occurs after peak of contraction
- Variable decelerations
  - Abrupt decrease in fetal heart rate with onset to nadir of less than 30 seconds
  - Nadir must be at least 15 beats per minute below the baseline and deceleration must last at least 15 seconds
- Prolonged decelerations
  - Decrease in fetal heart rate of at least 15 beats per minute below baseline
  - Lasts 2−10 minute

CLASSIFICATION OF FETAL HEART RATE TRACINGS[2,3,5]

Category I (Normal) (Fig. 8.3)

- Baseline rate: 110−160 beats per minute
- Baseline variability: moderate
- Accelerations: may be present or absent
- Early decelerations: may be present or absent
- Late/Variable decelerations: absent
- Interpretation: there is no fetal acidemia at that moment
- Management: continue routine fetal monitoring

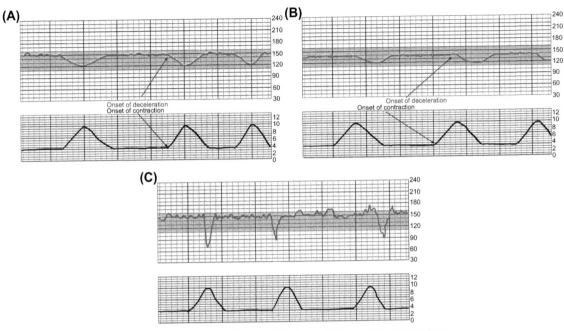

FIG. 8.2 Examples of **(A)** early, **(B)** late, and **(C)** variable decelerations.

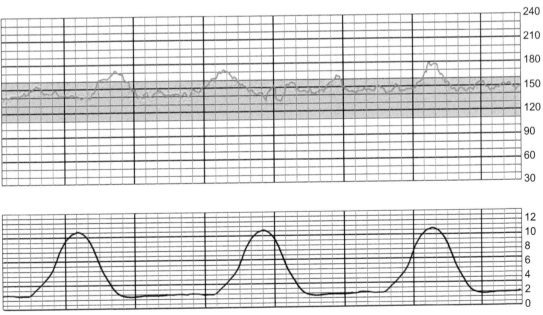

FIG. 8.3 Example of Category I fetal heart rate tracing. This tracing has a baseline of 145, moderate variability, accelerations, and no decelerations. Contractions are every 2.5–3 minutes.

Category II (Indeterminate) (Fig. 8.4)

- Includes everything not categorized as Category I or Category III. This may include any of the following:
  - Bradycardia without absent variability
  - Tachycardia
  - Prolonged deceleration
  - Minimal variability
  - Marked variability
  - Absent variability without recurrent decelerations
  - Moderated variability with recurrent late or variable decelerations
- Category II is not predictive of fetal acid—base status
- Management: continued evaluation and surveillance with intrauterine resuscitation measures as necessary; if intrauterine resuscitation fails to improve a fetal heart tracing with no accelerations and absent or minimal variability, consider delivery (Table 8.1)

Category III (Abnormal) (Fig. 8.5)

- Baseline variability absent AND any of the following:
  - Recurrent late decelerations
  - Recurrent variable decelerations
- Bradycardia
- Sinusoidal pattern (sine wave-like undulating pattern with a cycles frequency of 3—5 beats per minute that persists for 20 minutes or more)
- Associated with abnormal fetal acid—base status at the time observed
- Management:
  - Requires immediate intervention via intrauterine resuscitative measures and urgent delivery if intervention is ineffective

TABLE 8.1
Resuscitative Measures for Category II Tracing.

Recurrent late decelerations → reposition mother
Prolonged decelerations or bradycardia → oxygen
Minimal or absent variability → IV fluid bolus, reduce uterine contraction frequency
Recurrent variable decelerations → reposition mother, initiate amnioinfusion
Prolonged decelerations or bradycardia → check for cord prolapse

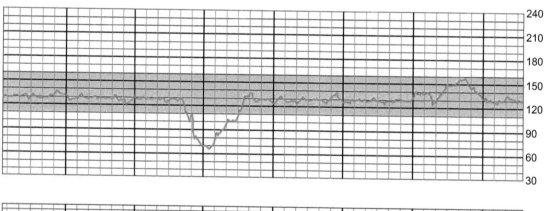

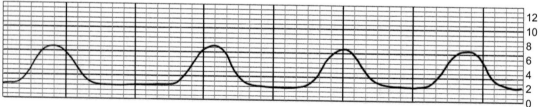

FIG. 8.4 Example of Category II fetal heart rate tracing. This tracing has a baseline of 130, moderate variability, an acceleration, and a variable deceleration. Contractions are every 2 minutes.

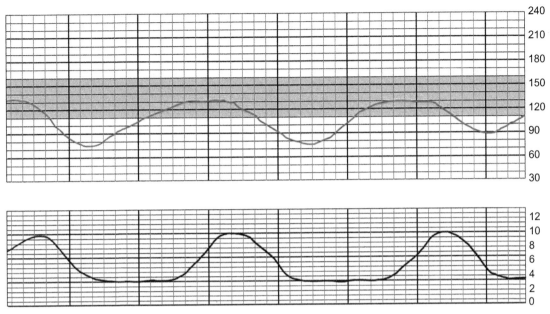

FIG. 8.5 Example of Category III fetal heart rate tracing. This tracing has a baseline of 140, absent variability, no accelerations, and recurrent late decelerations. Contractions are every 3 minutes.

UTERINE ACTIVITY MONITORING

Uterine activity monitoring is related to the quantification and description of uterine contractions. Assessment of uterine activity should be averaged over 30 minutes. It can be applied to spontaneous or induced labor.

- *Normal uterine activity* is five or fewer contractions in 10 minutes
- *Tachysystole* is greater than five contractions in 10 minutes. It is categorized by the presence or absence of decelerations (Fig. 8.6)
- Management of tachysystole depends on the category of tracing present. The management of tachysystole, as adapted from the American College of Obstetricians and Gynecologists, is summarized in Fig. 8.7[3]

LIMITATIONS OF FETAL HEART RATE MONITORING

Though now a part of routine obstetric care, fetal heart rate monitoring has not improved outcomes as originally hoped. Limitations of this technology include the following:

- Frequent false-positive tests (i.e., suspicion of fetal compromise when there is none) result in unnecessary surgical intervention
- No significant reduction in cerebral palsy or infant mortality

FETAL CORD GASES

The end goal of fetal heart rate monitoring is to improve fetal oxygen status. An objective measurement of this can be obtained after delivery by measuring fetal cord gases. The presence of normal gases virtually eliminates a diagnosis of severe intrapartum birth asphyxia. This measurement is reliable in both term and preterm infants.

General Interpretation of Fetal Cord Gases

- Arterial cord blood gas reflects **fetal** condition
- Venous cord blood gas reflects **placental** function

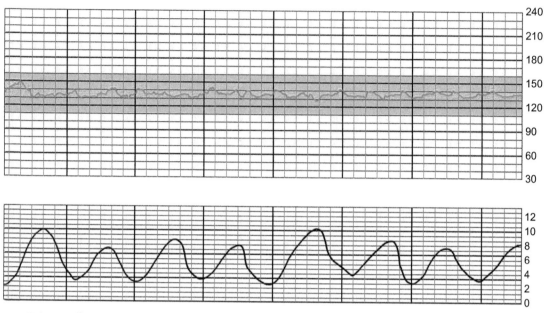

FIG. 8.6 Example of tachysystole without fetal heart rate changes. This tracing has a baseline of 135, moderate variability, no accelerations, and no decelerations. Contractions are every minute.

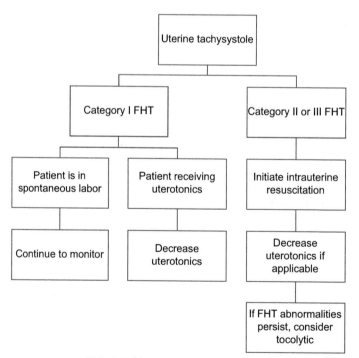

FIG. 8.7 Management of tachysystole.

TABLE 8.2
Normal cord gas values for term and preterm infants.

Acid-base factor	Preterm infants	Term infants
pH	7.29 ± 0.07	7.28 ± 0.07
pCO2 (mmHg)	49.2 ± 9.0	49.9 ± 14.2
pO2 (mmHg)	23.6 ± 8.9	23.7 ± 10.0
HCO3 (mmol/L)	23.0 ± 3.5	23.1 ± 2.8
Base deficit (mmol/L)	-3.3 ± 2.4	-3.6 ± 2.8

Reproduced from Ramin et al. 1989 with permission from Wolters Kluwer Health

- Normal gas results rule out the presence of acidemia at or immediately before delivery. Normal fetal cord gas values are listed in Table 8.2[6]

Management of Specific Fetal Cord Gas Abnormalities[7]

- Respiratory acidosis
  - Defined as:
    - Arterial pH < 7.20
    - Arterial PCO_2 >60
    - Base excess is > −2
  - Management: with stimulation and cry, baby will blow off excess CO_2
- Metabolic acidosis
  - Defined as:
    - Arterial pH < 7.20
    - Arterial PCO_2 <60
    - Base excess is < −2 to −9
  - Management: usually requires intensive resuscitation
  - Correlated with low APGAR scores and long-term neurologic deficits
- Metabolic acidemia
  - Defined as:
    - Arterial pH < 7.00
    - Base excess is ≤ −12

- Management: requires intensive resuscitation
- Correlated with hypoxic ischemic encephalopathy

REFERENCES

1. Caldeyro-Barcia R. *Control of the Human Fetal Heart Rate during Labor. The Heart and Circulation of the Newborn and Infant.* 1966:7−36.
2. American College of, O. and Gynecologists. ACOG practice bulletin No. 106: intrapartum fetal heart rate monitoring: nomenclature, interpretation, and general management principles. *Obstet Gynecol.* 2009;114(1):192−202.
3. American College of, O. and Gynecologists. Practice bulletin no. 116: management of intrapartum fetal heart rate tracings. *Obstet Gynecol.* 2010;116(5):1232−1240.
4. Macones GA, et al. The 2008 National Institute of Child Health and Human Development workshop report on electronic fetal monitoring: update on definitions, interpretation, and research guidelines. *Obstet Gynecol.* 2008;112(3):661−666.
5. Clark SL, et al. Intrapartum management of category II fetal heart rate tracings: towards standardization of care. *Am J Obstet Gynecol.* 2013;209(2):89−97.
6. Ramin SM, Gilstrap LC, Leveno KJ, Burris J, Little BB. Umbilical artery acid-base status in the preterm infant. *Obstet Gynecol.* 1989;74:256.
7. Pearson JF. Fetal blood sampling and gas exchange. *J Clin Pathol Suppl.* 1976;10:31−34.

Fetal Heart Tracing Simulation

MATERIALS NEEDED
- Copies of fetal heart rate tracing—this page may be reproduced for the purposes of simulation

KEY PERSONNEL
- Attending obstetrician
- Resident physician (if available in your institution)
- Nurse

SAMPLE SCENARIO
Patient is a 24-year-old G1P0 at 38 weeks who presents in active labor. Her initial cervical exam was 5/80/-2. Her FHT is as follows:

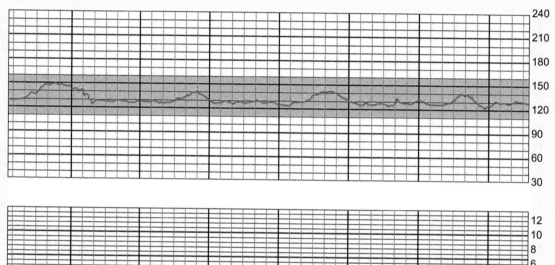

What is the best next step?

After 1 hour, patient's cervix is 6/90/-1. FHT is as follows:

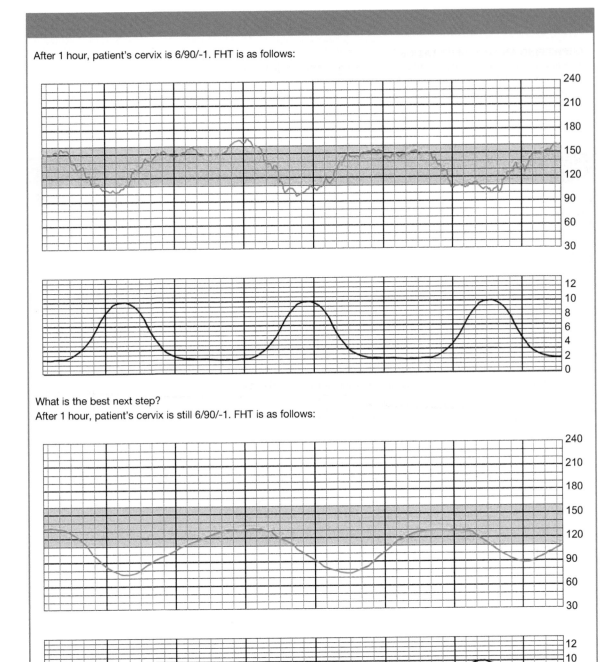

What is the best next step?

After 1 hour, patient's cervix is still 6/90/-1. FHT is as follows:

What is the best next step?

Continued

DEBRIEFING AND DOCUMENTATION
- Review interpretation of fetal heart rate tracings frequently with team members
- Document using three-tiered system (Category I, II, or III)
- Document intrauterine resuscitation strategies and fetal response to them

Simulation Checklist

		Time	Comments
Category I	Recognized reassuring nature of Category I tracing		
	Properly observed tracing		
Category II	Recognized uncertain nature of Category II tracing		
	Repositioned mother		
	Considered oxygen		
	Considered need to decrease uterotonics		
	Considered IV fluid bolus		
	Considered amnioinfusion		
Category III	Recognized concerning nature of Category III tracing		
	Proceeded with delivery		

Technical Skills	Non-Technical Skills
Understand standard nomenclature to describe fetal heart rate tracings	Recognize clinical context of abnormal fetal heart rate tracings
List interventions for abnormal fetal heart rate tracings	Communicate with team members
List interventions for tachysystole	Communicate with patient

Let's debrief. . .

Technical and nontechnical skills for fetal heart rate monitoring.

Shoulder Dystocia

Shoulder dystocia is an obstetric emergency. It occurs when, following delivery of the fetal head, routine gentle traction fails to deliver the fetal shoulders.[1]

RISK FACTORS

Known risk factors for shoulder dystocia include:

- High birth weight
- Diabetes mellitus
- Previous shoulder dystocia
- Postterm pregnancy
- Abnormal labor progress
- Operative vaginal delivery
- Male fetal gender
- Maternal obesity and high gestational weight gain
- Advanced maternal age
- African-American

Most shoulder dystocia cases occur in women with no risk factors. The obstetric team must be prepared for the possibility of shoulder dystocia with every delivery.

PREVENTION OF SHOULDER DYSTOCIA

Scheduled cesarean delivery is reasonable in the following cases:

- Prior shoulder dystocia, especially with a severe neonatal injury
- Estimated fetal weight >4500 g in women with diabetes (estimated risk of shoulder dystocia 15%)
- Estimated fetal weight >5000 g in women without diabetes (estimated risk of shoulder dystocia >20%)

In addition, women with estimated fetal weights >4000 g who undergo a trial of labor become high risk for shoulder intrapartum if they have a prolonged second stage or require an operative vaginal delivery.[2]

DIAGNOSIS

Shoulder dystocia is a subjective clinical diagnosis. During delivery of the fetal head, difficulty with birth of the face and chin may be present. When the head of the infant is born, it remains tightly applied to the vulva. In addition, the "turtle sign" or retraction of the fetal head against the maternal perineum may be present.

Difficulty or failure to accomplish external rotation of the head after it has passed the perineum is another sign suggestive of shoulder dystocia. Finally, resistance to the delivery of the anterior shoulder with the usual amount of traction applied to the fetal head should alert the delivering provider of the diagnosis of shoulder dystocia.

MANAGEMENT

Initial Steps

- CALL FOR HELP!! Personnel in the delivery room should include:

  - An experienced care provider
  - Two labor and delivery nurses
  - A neonatologist
  - An anesthesiologist

Safety Training for Obstetric Emergencies. https://doi.org/10.1016/B978-0-323-69672-2.00009-6

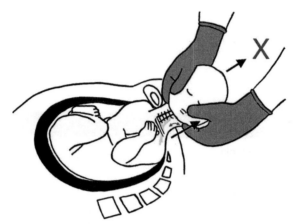

FIG. 9.1 Avoid traction on fetal neck during delivery as this can result in brachial plexus injury.

- State clearly "There is a shoulder dystocia."
- Explain to patient the presence of shoulder dystocia and the need for additional maneuvers
- Position the patient with her buttocks at the edge of the bed, lower the bed, and request a stool to assist with specific maneuvers
- Note the time the head was delivered (START THE CLOCK)
- Evaluate the need for episiotomy. This will not relieve the shoulder dystocia but will allow more room for performing maneuvers
- If the bladder is distended, drain it
- Avoid excessive head and neck traction (Fig. 9.1)
- If a tight nuchal cord is encountered, release the cord if possible; avoid clamping and cutting the cord
- NEVER apply fundal pressure. This can further engage the anterior shoulder under the pubic bone
- Implement maneuvers to alleviate shoulder dystocia. Move quickly between maneuvers and do not persist in any one maneuver if it is not immediately successful

McRoberts' Maneuver[3,4]

- Requires two assistants who each support a maternal leg and flex the thigh sharply against the abdomen
- Causes cephalad displacement of the symphysis, flattens the sacral promontory, and improves pushing efficiency
- Often recommended as initial or even prophylactic maneuver due to its low invasiveness

- There is not an order for the other maneuvers. The preference is given to the experience of the operator.

Suprapubic Pressure

- An assistant applies suprapubic pressure with his/her palm or fist. It is crucial that pressure is applied suprapubic, *not fundal*
- Pressure is applied in a downward (below pubic bone) and lateral direction (toward the baby face or sternum) to decrease the bisacromial diameter and shift this diameter into an oblique position
- This maneuver is performed simultaneously with McRoberts' maneuver (Fig. 9.2)

Delivery of the Posterior Arm (Jacquemier's Maneuver)[5,6]

- Highly effective maneuver to relieve anterior shoulder impaction
- It is best performed under adequate anesthesia
- The provider passes a hand into the vagina over the chest of the fetus to identify the posterior arm and elbow
- If the fetal chest faces the maternal right, then the operator introduces the left hand and vice versa
- Pressure is applied to the antecubital fossa and the elbow is flexed in front of the body, and/or the posterior hand is grasped to sweep the arm across the chest and deliver the arm. Avoid applying pressure directly to the humeral shaft to reduce the risk of fracture
- The fetus is rotated into the oblique diameter of the pelvis, bringing the anterior shoulder under the symphysis pubis (Fig. 9.3)

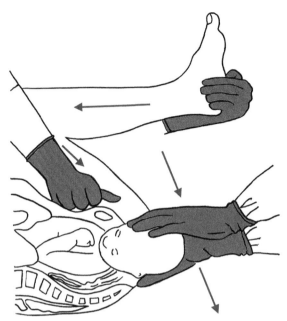

FIG. 9.2 McRoberts' maneuver and suprapubic pressure. Hips are flexed to flatten the sacral promontory. Suprapubic pressure decreases the bisacromial diameter. Together, these improve pushing efficiency.

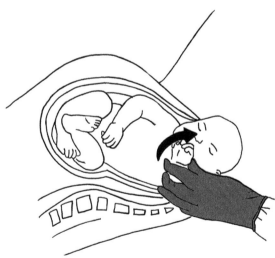

FIG. 9.3 Jacquemier's maneuver. The posterior arm is swept over the fetal chest and delivered.

Rubin Maneuver[7]

- The operator places a hand on the back surface of the posterior shoulder (right hand if the fetal chest is facing the maternal right and vice versa)

- If the anterior shoulder is more accessible, the hand can be placed in the back of the anterior shoulder
- Pressure causes adduction of the fetal shoulder and allows displacement of the bisacromial diameter from the anteroposterior position to the oblique position (Fig. 9.4)

Woods' Screw Maneuver[8]

- Pressure is applied on the anterior (clavicular) surface of the posterior shoulder (Fig. 9.5A)
- The fetus is rotated 180° until the formerly posterior shoulder is now anterior and has passed under the pubic symphysis
- Pressure is now applied to the posterior surface of the anterior shoulder (Fig. 9.5B) to rotate the fetus 180° in the opposite direction. This effects delivery of the second shoulder (Fig. 9.5C)

Delivery of the Posterior Shoulder (Menticoglou Maneuver)[9,10]

- This maneuver is used when it is not possible to reach the elbow or forearm because the posterior arm is above the pelvic brim
- An assistant gently flexes the fetal head toward the anterior shoulder
- The operator places the right middle finger into the fetus' posterior axilla from the left side of the pelvis and the left middle finger into the posterior axilla from the right side of the pelvis
- This middle finger "hook" is used to bring the posterior shoulder down along the curvature of the sacrum (Fig. 9.6). This may dislodge the anterior shoulder or allow the posterior arm to be delivered with the maneuver described earlier

Gaskin Maneuver[11]

- The patient is moved to an all fours position with her back arched
- This position increases the space in the hollow of the sacrum and allows gravity to facilitate delivery
- Gentle downward traction of the shoulder against the maternal sacrum or upward traction of the shoulder next to the symphysis is applied (Fig. 9.7)

Clavicular Fracture[12]

- Intentional fracture of the clavicle may shorten the bisacromial diameter
- The anterior clavicle is grasped and pulled outward

(A)

(B)

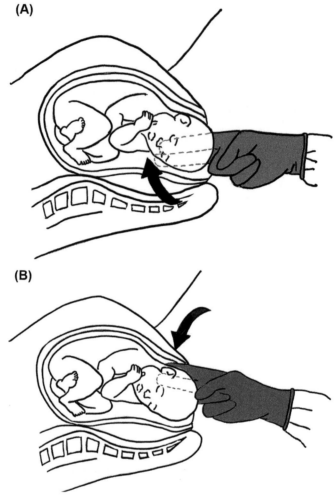

FIG. 9.4 Rubin maneuver. Pressure applied to the posterior aspect of the fetal shoulder causes adduction and a decreased bisacromial diameter. Pressure may be applied to **(A)** posterior or **(B)** anterior shoulder.

- It can be a difficult procedure and it can cause injury of underlying neurovascular and pulmonary structures. Despite this, it is typically less morbid than the procedures of last resort

LAST RESORT MANEUVERS
Abdominal Rescue

- When the classical maneuvers are unsuccessful, transabdominal fetal rotation of the anterior shoulder may be attempted through a hysterotomy

- The abdomen is entered for a cesarean delivery, and transabdominal pressure is used to dislodge the impacted fetal shoulder
- Vaginal delivery is attempted

Gunn-Zavanelli-O'Leary Maneuver[13,14]

- Relax the uterus
  - Terbutaline 0.25 mg subcutaneously
  - *OR* nitroglycerin 50–500 mcg intravenously in aliquots of 50–100 mcg

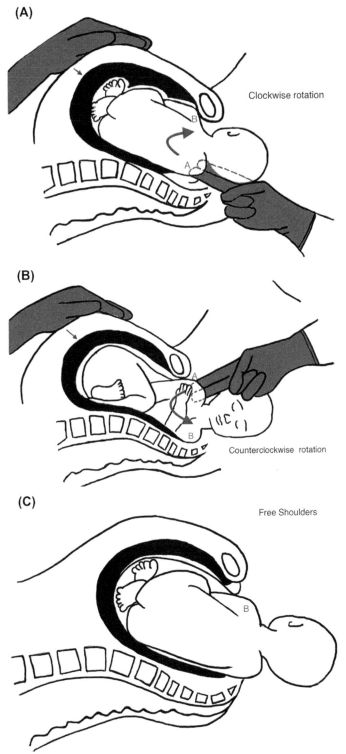

(A)

Clockwise rotation

(B)

Counterclockwise rotation

(C)

Free Shoulders

FIG. 9.5 Woods' screw maneuver. **(A)** Pressure applied to the anterior aspect of the posterior fetal shoulder causes rotation of the fetus and dislodgement of the first shoulder. **(B)** The fetus is then rotated in the opposite direction to **(C)** deliver the remaining shoulder.

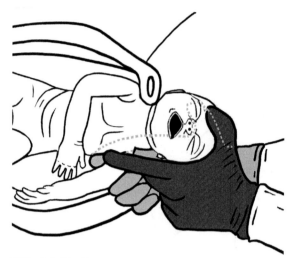

FIG. 9.6 Modified Menticoglou maneuver. The posterior shoulder is brought along the curvature of the sacrum.

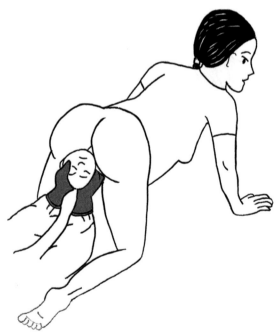

FIG. 9.7 Gaskin maneuver. The mother is rotated to all fours and delivery maneuvers are reattempted.

- Rotate the head back to an occiput anterior position (reversal of cardinal movements)
- Flex the head and push as far as possible in a vertical/cephalad axis
- If successful, perform a cesarean delivery (Fig. 9.8)

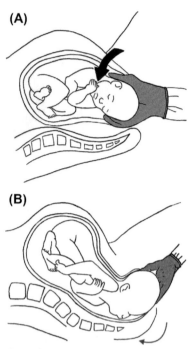

(A)

(B)

FIG. 9.8 Gunn-Zavanelli-O'Leary maneuver. The fetal head is pushed back into the uterus by reversing the cardinal movements of labor and a cesarean delivery is performed.

Symphysiotomy[15]

- Perform only as a last resort if operating room not available
- Infiltrate skin over symphysis pubis with local anesthetic
- Place the index finger of the nondominant hand transvaginally to displace the urethra from the midline
- Create a small skin incision over the symphysis pubis
- Incise the cartilaginous portion of the pubic symphysis just deep enough to allow modest separation
- While symphysiotomy carries a high complication rate (including injury to the genitourinary tract, vesical incontinence, fistulas, long term pain, and pelvic instability), it may be lifesaving (Fig. 9.9)

COMPLICATIONS[1]
Fetal Complications

- Brachial plexus palsy (may be transient or permanent)
- Clavicular fracture

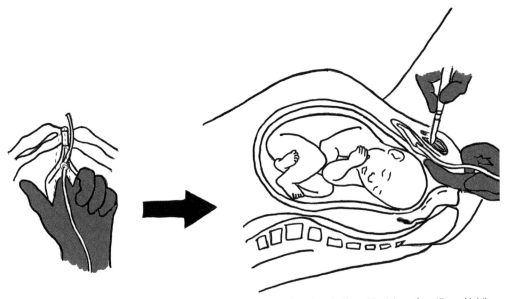

FIG. 9.9 Symphysiotomy. Diagram shows displacement of urethra (left) and incision of cartilage (right).

- Humerus fracture
- Hypoxic ischemic encephalopathy
- Death

Maternal Complications

- Postpartum hemorrhage
- Pelvic floor injuries
- Symphyseal separation
- Lateral femoral cutaneous neuropathy
- Urethral injury
- Bladder injury
- Uterine rupture

REFERENCES

1. Committee on Practice B-O. Practice bulletin No 178: shoulder dystocia. *Obstet Gynecol.* 2017;129(5): e123–e133.
2. Herzberg S, Kabiri D, Mordechai T, et al. Fetal macrosomia as a risk factor for shoulder dystocia during vacuum extraction. *J Matern Fetal Neonatal Med.* 2017;30(15): 1870–1873.
3. Gherman RB, Chauhan S, Ouzounian JG, Lerner H, Gonik B, Goodwin TM. Shoulder dystocia: the unpreventable obstetric emergency with empiric management guidelines. *Am J Obstet Gynecol.* 2006;195(3):657–672.
4. McRoberts WJCOG. Maneuvers for shoulder dystocia. *Contemp Obstet Gynecol.* 1984;24:17.
5. Maggiora-Vergano T. The Jacquemier-Varnier maneuver as treatment of shoulder dystocia in birth by the cephalic extremity. *La Clinica ostetrica e ginecologica.* 1961;63:31–34.
6. Barnum CG. Dystocia due to the shoulders. *Am J Obstet Gynecol.* 1945;50(4):439–442.
7. Rubin A. Management of shoulder dystocia. *JAMA.* 1964; 189:835–837.
8. Woods CE. A principle of physics as applicable to shoulder delivery. *Am J Obstet Gynecol.* 1943;45(5):796–804.
9. Gilstrop M, Hoffman MK. An update on the acute management of shoulder dystocia. *Clin Obstet Gynecol.* 2016;59(4):813–819.
10. Menticoglou SMJO. A modified technique to deliver the posterior arm in severe shoulder dystocia. *Obstet Gynecol.* 2006;108(3):755–757.
11. Bruner JP, Drummond SB, Meenan AL, Gaskin IM. All-fours maneuver for reducing shoulder dystocia during labor. *J Reprod Med.* 1998;43(5):439–443.
12. Joseph PR, Rosenfeld W. Clavicular fractures in neonates. *Am J Dis Child.* 1990;144(2):165–167.
13. O'Leary JA, Gunn D. Cephalic replacement for shoulder dystocia. *Am J Obstet Gynecol.* 1985;153(5):592.
14. Sandberg EC. The Zavanelli maneuver: a potentially revolutionary method for the resolution of shoulder dystocia. *Am J Obstet Gynecol.* 1985;152(4):479–484.
15. Smyly WJ. A case of symphysiotomy. *Br Med J.* 1893; 1(1687):885.

Shoulder Dystocia Simulation

MATERIALS NEEDED
- Model of pelvis
- Fetal manikin

KEY PERSONNEL
- Anesthesiologist
- Attending obstetrician
- Neonatologist
- Resident physician (if available in your institution)
- Two nurses

SAMPLE SCENARIO

Jolene is a 36-year-old G1P0 at 40 weeks 4 days gestation presented in labor. She had a prolonged active phase and required Pitocin augmentation. She began pushing approximately 2.5 hours ago and has been making progress. Pregnancy was complicated by hypothyroidism and gestational diabetes. Estimated fetal weight by Leopold's is 9#. The head is beginning to crown and the team is assembled for delivery.

After the head delivers, it retracts against the perineum. The delivering physician recognizes a shoulder dystocia.

DEBRIEFING AND DOCUMENTATION
- Estimated fetal weight prior to delivery
- Risk factors for shoulder dystocia
- Preparatory measures for potential shoulder dystocia
  - Position of bed
  - Communication with family
- Time for delivery of head to body
- Maneuver sequence
- Which arm delivered first
- Was an episiotomy performed? (and if so, was it before or after delivery of the head)
- Blood loss at delivery
- Description of maternal and/or neonatal injuries
- Communication with patient and family

Simulation Checklist		Time	Comments
Initial response	Recognized shoulder dystocia		
	Called for help		
	Communicated clearly "we have a shoulder dystocia."		
Maneuvers	McRoberts		
	Suprapubic pressure		
	Woods' screw		
	Rubin's		
	Posterior arm delivery		
	Gaskin (all-fours)		
	Clavicular fracture		
	Zavanelli		
Documentation	Timing of delivery of head, body		
	Which shoulder was anterior		
	Maneuvers used		
	Infant birthweight		
	APGAR scores		
	Infant moving all extremities		
	Persons present		
	Blood loss		
Communication	Kept patient and partner informed		
	Call-out		
	Directed communication		
	Closed-loop communication		

Technical Skills	Non-Technical Skills
List risk factors for shoulder dystocia	Use call-out communication
Perform maneuvers for shoulder dystocia	Call for help
List maternal complications from shoulder dystocia	Communicate with patient
List fetal complications from shoulder dystocia	Debrief with team

Let's debrief. . .

Technical and nontechnical skills for shoulder dystocia.

Operative Vaginal Delivery

Operative vaginal delivery is a delivery in which the operator uses forceps or a vacuum to facilitate the delivery of the fetus. When successful, operative vaginal delivery avoids cesarean delivery and all the associated morbidities and complications. It should be performed *only* by experienced obstetricians and care providers with privileges.

INDICATIONS FOR OPERATIVE VAGINAL DELIVERY[1]

- Prolonged second stage of labor
- Suspicion of immediate or potential fetal compromise
- Shortening of the second stage of labor for maternal benefit (e.g., cardiac, neurologic, or lung disease)

CONTRAINDICATIONS TO OPERATIVE VAGINAL DELIVERY[1]

- Unengaged head
- Unknown position of fetal head
- Live fetus with known or strongly suspected bone demineralization disorder or bleeding disorder
- Brow or face presentation
- Suspected fetal–pelvic disproportion

VACUUM-ASSISTED VAGINAL DELIVERY

Vacuum-assisted delivery (Fig. 10.1) has risen in popularity largely due to a belief that it is easier to learn. It is generally less traumatic for the mother than forceps-assisted delivery. However, it still carries a risk of neonatal complications and should only be used by skilled providers. It is more likely to fail than forceps-

assisted delivery.[2] Use of vacuum under 34 weeks of gestation or in small fetuses is discouraged[1].

Vacuum Extraction Technique[3-5]

- Obtain maternal consent to proceed with operative vaginal delivery
- Confirm the bladder is empty, the cervix is fully dilated, and fetal position is known
- Test for proper function of the vacuum equipment
- Identify the flexion point 3 cm anterior to the posterior fontanelle and centered over the sagittal suture (Fig. 10.2)
- Place the vacuum cup over the flexion point while ensuring that there is no maternal tissue under the cup
- Initiate vacuum pressure according to the manufacturer instructions (typically 450–600 mmHg) (Fig. 10.3)

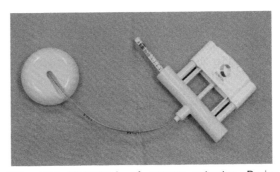

FIG. 10.1 Photograph of vacuum extractor. Device pictured is Kiwi complete vacuum delivery system by Clinical Innovations.

Safety Training for Obstetric Emergencies. https://doi.org/10.1016/B978-0-323-69672-2.00010-2

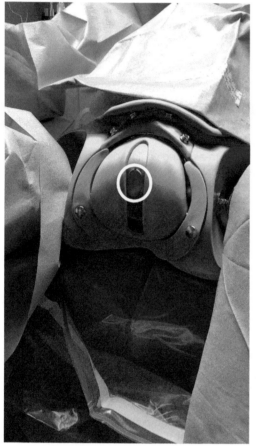

FIG. 10.2 The center of the vacuum cup should be placed at flexion point, which is 3 cm anterior to the posterior fontanelle. In most babies, this will mean the edge of the cup will be 3 cm posterior to the anterior fontanelle.

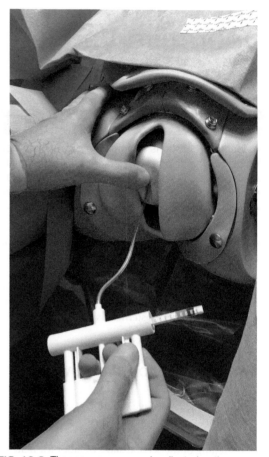

FIG. 10.3 The vacuum pressure is adjusted so the pressure is in the "green zone" as labeled by the manufacturer, typically 450–600 mmHg.

- With each contraction, apply traction in the direction of the pelvic curvature (Fig. 10.4). Do NOT employ rocking motions or rotational force
- Consider abandoning attempt at operative vaginal delivery if any of the following occurs[5]:
  - No progress in one to two pulls
  - Delivery is not imminent after four contractions and/or 20 minutes
  - There are three pop-offs without an obvious cause

FORCEPS-ASSISTED VAGINAL DELIVERY[6]

Forceps delivery is more likely than vacuum to result in a successful vaginal birth. It allows the operator to rotate the fetus. However, it is more likely to result in

third and fourth perineal tears than is vacuum-assisted delivery. "Baby" Elliot and "baby" Simpson forceps[7] have been used for small fetuses. We suggest avoiding forceps for fetuses under 1500 g of weight. We suggest becoming familiar with one type of forceps. We prefer the Simpson forceps (Fig. 10.5).

Types of Forceps Deliveries[1]

- Outlet forceps
  - Scalp is visible at the introitus without separating the labia
  - Fetal skull has reached the pelvic floor
  - Fetal head is at or on perineum
  - Sagittal suture is in anteroposterior diameter or right or left occiput anterior or posterior position
  - Rotation does not exceed 45°

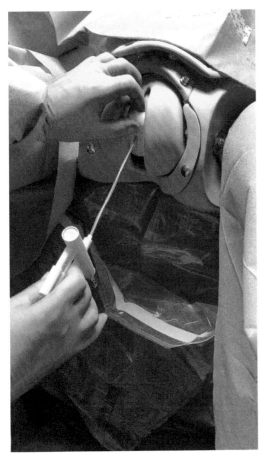

FIG. 10.4 Traction is applied in a J-like motion following the direction of the pelvic curvature.

- Low forceps
  - Leading point at the fetal skull is at station +2 cm or more and not on the pelvic floor
  - If rotation is greater than 45°, classified as "low forceps with rotation"

- Midforceps
  - Station is above +2 cm but head is engaged

Forceps Delivery Technique[8]

- Obtain maternal consent to proceed with operative vaginal delivery
- Confirm the bladder is empty, the cervix is fully dilated, and fetal position can be assessed
- Perform a "phantom application" with the forceps blades. Visualize how the blades would appear when correctly applied. Begin with a delicate hold of the left blade in the left hand. Then, apply the right blade on top of the left and lock together
- Apply forceps to fetal head between contractions. Again, apply the left blade followed by the right blade and ensure they are locked in place (Fig. 10.6)
- If the right blade is placed first, the blades will not properly lock in place. The operator must first separate the blade and rotate the right blade up and over the left blade (Fig. 10.7).
- The following safety checks should be performed to assure that forceps are appropriately placed:
  - The sagittal suture should be aligned with the shanks
  - The posterior fontanelle should be one finger breath above the shanks
  - The lambdoid sutures should be equidistant for the forceps blades
  - The fenestrated blades should admit no more than one finger breadth between the heel of the fenestration and the fetal head
  - No maternal tissue should be grasped
- Consider abandoning attempt at operative vaginal delivery if any of the following occur:
  - There is failure of proper application
  - There is failure of attempted rotation
  - There is inadequate descent with traction

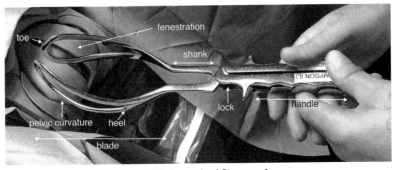

FIG. 10.5 Photograph of Simpson forceps.

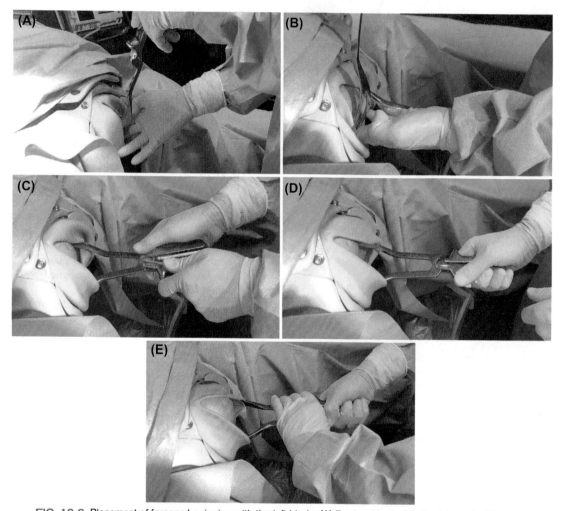

FIG. 10.6 Placement of forceps beginning with the left blade. **(A)** Begin with placing the left blade. **(B)** Then, place the right blade. **(C)** The blades will fit easily together and **(D)** lock in place. **(E)** Traction is then placed in the direction of the maternal pelvis to effect delivery.

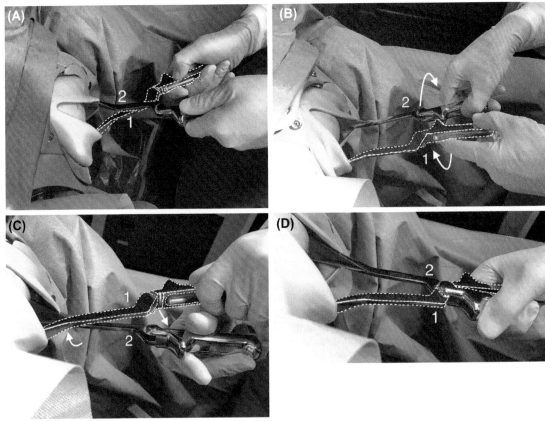

FIG. 10.7 Placement of the forceps beginning with the right blade. **(A)** The blades will not lock together if the right blade is below the left blade. **(B)** The blades are separated. **(C)** The right blade is rotated clockwise over the left blade. **(D)** This will allow proper locking of the blades.

COMPLICATIONS OF OPERATIVE VAGINAL DELIVERY

Fetal Complications

- Scalp trauma (hemorrhage, laceration)
- Subgaleal hemorrhage
- Skull fracture
- Facial nerve palsy
- Hyperbilirubinemia
- Retinal hemorrhage

Maternal Complications

- Third and fourth degree laceration
- Vaginal hematoma

REFERENCES

1. Committee on Practice B-O. ACOG practice bulletin No. 154: operative vaginal delivery. *Obstet Gynecol.* 2015; 126(5):e56–65.
2. O'Mahony F, Hofmeyr GJ, Menon V. Choice of instruments for assisted vaginal delivery. *Cochrane Database of Syst Rev.* 2010;(11). Art. No.: CD005455. https://doi.org/10.1002/14651858.CD005455.pub2.
3. Vacca A. Vacuum-assisted delivery. *Best Pract Res Clin Obstet Gynaecol.* 2002;16(1):17–30.
4. Murphy DJ, Liebling RE, Patel R, Verity L, Swingler R. Cohort study of operative delivery in the second stage of labour and standard of obstetric care. *BJOG.* 2003;110(6):610–615.
5. Clinical Innovations. Complete Vacuum Delivery System with PalmPump; 2018. Available from http://clinicalinnovations.com/wp-content.
6. Hale RW. *Dennen's Forceps Deliveries: American College of Obstetricians and Gynecologists Women's Health Care Physicians.* 2001.
7. Simpson ARJE. On axis-traction forceps. *Edinb Med J.* 1880; 26(4):289.
8. Simpson AN, Gurau D, Secter M, et al. Learning from experience: development of a cognitive task list to Perform a safe and successful non-rotational forceps delivery. *J Obstet Gynaecol Can.* 2015;37(7):589–597.

Vacuum-Assisted Delivery Simulation

MATERIALS NEEDED
- Model of pelvis
- Fetal manikin
- Vacuum extractor
- Forceps (Simpson)

KEY PERSONNEL
- Attending obstetrician
- Neonatologist
- Nurse
- Resident physician (if available in your institution)

SAMPLE SCENARIO

A 22-year-old G1P0 at 38 weeks 5 days presented in active labor. On initial exam, her cervix was 5 cm dilated, 80% effaced, and −2 station. Estimated fetal weight is approximately seven pounds. She received an epidural and progressed through an uncomplicated labor. She is now fully dilated and has been pushing for 2 hours with good descent of the head. She states that she is exhausted and cannot push anymore. The head is at +3 station. She asks if there is anything you can do to help her.

DEBRIEFING AND DOCUMENTATION
- Indication for operative vaginal delivery
- Amount of molding and caput present
- Adequacy of maternal pelvis
- Instrument used
- Prerequisites fulfilled
- Fetal position and station
- Number of pulls
- Number of pop-offs
- Description of maternal and/or neonatal injuries
- Communication with patient and family

Simulation Checklist

		Time	Comments
Safe vacuum steps	Ensured patient had adequate anesthesia		
	Emptied bladder		
	Confirmed cervix fully dilated, membranes ruptured		
	Determined fetal position		
	Inspected and tested vacuum or Forceps		
	Identified flexion point		
	Cup placed on flexion point		
	Provided gentle traction		
	Stopped attempts if: • No progress in 1–2 pulls • Delivery not imminent after four contractions and/or 20 minutes • Three pop-offs without an obvious cause		
	Considered need for episiotomy		
	Removed vacuum after jaw reachable		
	Anticipated shoulder dystocia		
Documentation	Indication for operative vaginal delivery		
	Adequacy of pelvis		
	Instrument used		
	Fetal position and station		
	Number of pulls		
	Number of pop-offs		
	Description of maternal and/or neonatal injuries		
Communication	Called for help		
	Obtained consent from patient		
	Completed debriefing with patient		

Technical Skills	Non-Technical Skills
List contraindications to operative vaginal delivery	Prepare for complications of operative vaginal delivery
Apply vacuum correctly	Call for help
Apply forceps correctly	Communicate with family
Demonstrate proper operative vaginal delivery technique	Debrief with team

Technical and nontechnical skills for operative vaginal delivery.

Vaginal Breech Delivery

Breech presentation occurs when the presenting part of the fetus is the buttocks or feet. There are three main types of breech presentation Fig. 11.1.

TYPES OF VAGINAL BREECH DELIVERY

- Spontaneous breech delivery → fetus delivers without assistance or manipulation; usually occurs when fetus is preterm
- Assisted breech delivery → fetus descends with a "hands-off" approach. Recognized maneuvers are used to assist when required

- Breech extraction → one or both fetal feet are grasped from the uterine cavity and brought down through the vagina; usually reserved for delivery of a second twin

MANAGEMENT

Optimal Patient Selection[1,2]

- No contraindication to vaginal birth
- No prior cesarean deliveries
- Gestational age >36 weeks
- Spontaneous labor

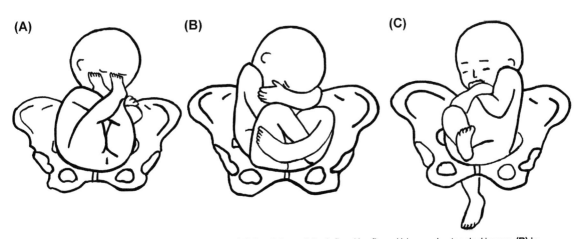

(A) **(B)** **(C)**

FIG. 11.1 Types of breech presentation. **(A)** Frank breech is defined by flexed hips and extended knees. **(B)** In complete breech, the fetus has flexed hips and flexed knees. **(C)** In incomplete breech, there is extension of at least one of the fetal hips.

- Facility equipped for safe emergency cesarean delivery
- Staff skilled in breech delivery
- Ultrasound examination showing:
  - Frank or complete breech presentation
  - No hyperextension of the fetal head
  - Absence of any fetal anomaly that may cause dystocia
  - Estimated fetal weight between 2000 and 3500 g
  - Incomplete breech presentation is a contraindication to vaginal delivery (high risk of cord prolapse)

Labor Management[2]

- Avoid induction of labor
- Determine the type of breech (ultrasound and/or physical examination)
- Avoid artificial rupture of membranes. Perform vaginal exam after spontaneous rupture of membranes to exclude cord prolapse
- Continuous electronic fetal monitoring—if necessary, place fetal scalp electrode on buttocks
- Consider regional anesthesia
- In case of poor labor progress in the active phase, cesarean delivery should be considered. Data suggests better outcomes if the second stage is less than 40 minutes[3]

Delivery Technique[4-6]

- Dorsal lithotomy or any other "upright" maternal positions are acceptable options
- Empty the bladder and remove any indwelling catheter
- Perform episiotomy only if necessary and not until the presenting part is at the level of the vulva
- Once the breech is visible at the perineum, encourage active pushing
- The mother bears down until feet, legs, and trunk to the scapula are visible. Spontaneous delivery of the limbs and trunk is preferable—do not pull! (Fig. 11.2)
- If the legs are extended after the umbilicus has delivered, legs may be delivered by Pinard maneuver, which employs a constant pressure on the back of the knee (Fig. 11.3)
- Check cord pulsation and pull a small loop of cord down to prevent traction on the cord

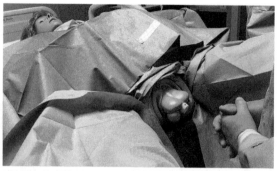

FIG. 11.2 Encourage active pushing keeping the hands off.

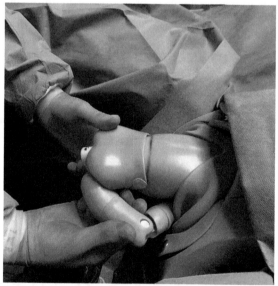

FIG. 11.3 Pinard maneuver. Pressure is exerted on the back of the knee. This assists delivery of extended legs.

- If the arms do not deliver spontaneously, support the fetus by placing your hands at the levels of the bony prominences of the iliac crests (Fig. 11.4)
- Rotate the fetus 180° to deliver the first shoulder and arm. Then, repeat in the opposite direction. This is called Løvset's maneuver (Fig. 11.5)

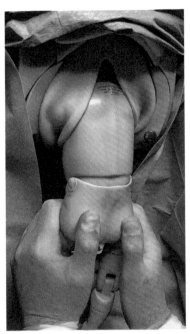

FIG. 11.4 The practitioner's hands are placed on the bony prominences of the iliac crests.

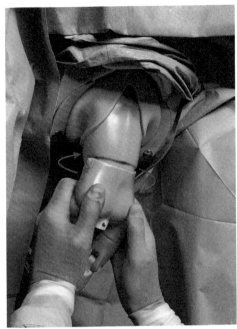

FIG. 11.5 Løvset's maneuver. The fetal body is supported and rotated from side to side to allow delivery of arms. Note location of supporting hands on bony prominences of iliac crests to limit potential for internal soft tissue injury.

- Failure to deliver the arms with simple rotation may indicate the need to assist by sliding an index finger along the fetal scapula, over the shoulder, and into the antecubital fossa. The elbow is then swept in front of the face and downward to the chest. This procedure is repeated on the other side (Fig. 11.6)
- After delivery of the arms, have an assistant apply suprapubic pressure and deliver the head by simultaneously supporting the legs and directing the fetal body axis upwards (Modified Bracht maneuver; Fig. 11.7).
- In the case of a difficult head delivery, the following techniques may be useful[7-11]:
  - Piper forceps[9] (Fig. 11.8)—An assistant holds the body of the fetus. Piper forceps are applied underneath the fetal body. The axis of traction aims to flex the fetal head (Fig. 11.9)

- Mauriceau–Smellie–Veit maneuver—The baby's body is supported on the flexor surface of the practitioner's forearm
  The first and third fingers of the supporting hand are placed on the cheekbones and the other hand applies pressure to the fetal occiput (Fig. 11.10). If the cervix constricts the fetal head, the first step is administration of nitroglycerine IV (100 mcg/IV)
- Burns–Marshall technique—The fetal body is raised vertically while an assistant holds the baby's feet
- Dührssen's incisions—If the head remains entrapped in the cervix, particularly in a preterm delivery, the cervix can be incised to release the head. Incisions are made at 2, 6, and 10 o'clock positions to avoid neurovascular bundles (Fig. 11.11)

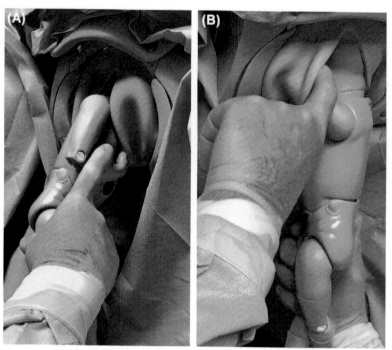

FIG. 11.6 Manual delivery of fetal arms. **(A)** The practitioner slides an index finger along the fetal scapula, over the shoulder, and into the antecubital fossa. The right upper extremity is delivered **(B)** The fetus is rotated 180 degree s and the process is repeated for the left upper extrenity.

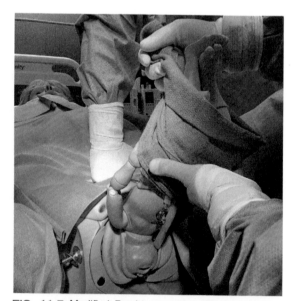

FIG. 11.7 Modified Bracht maneuver. The fetal head is delivered with suprapubic pressure and elevation of the body.

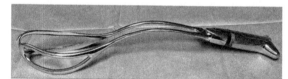

FIG. 11.8 Piper forceps are used to aid delivery of the fetal head.

FETAL COMPLICATIONS

- Intrapartum death
- Intracranial hemorrhage
- Hypoxic ischemic encephalopathy
- Brachial plexus injury
- Rupture of the liver, kidney, or spleen
- Dislocation of the neck, shoulder, or hip
- Fractured clavicle, humerus, or femur
- Cord prolapse

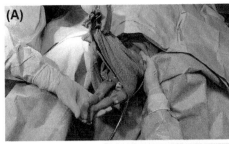

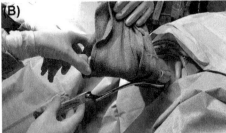

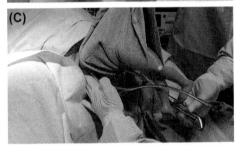

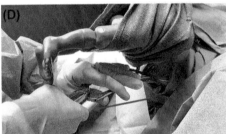

FIG. 11.9 Piper forceps technique. **(A)** The body is elevated and the left blade is placed. **(B)** Proper placement of the blade is below the fetal body. **(C)** The right blade is placed in a similar manner. **(D)** Traction is placed in line with the maternal pelvis to facilitate head flexion.

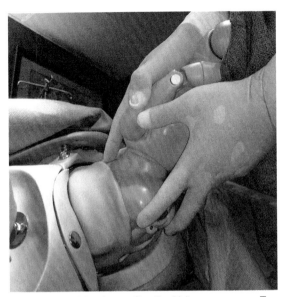

FIG. 11.10 Mauriceau–Smellie–Veit maneuver. Two fingers of the dominant hand are applied to the fetal cheekbones to aid head flexion.

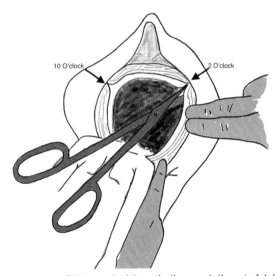

FIG. 11.11 Dührssen incisions. In the event, there is fetal head entrapment in the cervix, the cervix can be incised at the 2, 6, and 10 o'clock positions.

REFERENCES

1. Practice ACoO. ACOG Committee Opinion No. 340. Mode of term singleton breech delivery. *Obstet Gynecol.* 2006;108(1):235−237.
2. Kotaska A, Menticoglou S, Gagnon R, et al. SOGC clinical practice guideline: vaginal delivery of breech presentation: no. 226, June 2009. *Int J Gynaecol Obstet.* 2009;107(2):169−176.
3. Macharey G, Ulander VM, Heinonen S, Kostev K, Nuutila M, Väisänen-Tommiska M. Risk factors and outcomes in "well-selected" vaginal breech deliveries: a retrospective observational study. *J Perinat Med.* 2017;45(3):291−297.
4. Secter MB, Simpson AN, Gurau D, et al. Learning from experience: qualitative analysis to develop a cognitive task list for vaginal breech deliveries. *J Obstet Gynaecol Can.* 2015;37(11):966−974.
5. Louwen F, Daviss BA, Johnson KC, Reitter A. Does breech delivery in an upright position instead of on the back improve outcomes and avoid cesareans? *Int J Gynaecol Obstet.* 2017;136(2):151−161.
6. Heres MH, Pel M, Elferink-Stinkens PM, Van Hemel OJ, Treffers PE. The Dutch obstetric intervention study–variations in practice patterns. *Int J Gynaecol Obstet.* 1995;50(2):145−150.
7. Plentl AA, Stone RE. The bracht maneuver. *J Obstetr Gynecol Survey.* 1953;8(3):313−325.
8. Dührssen A. Ueber den Werth der tiefen Cervix-und Scheiden-Damm[-Einschnitte in der Geburtshülfe. *Arch Gynäkol.* 1890;37(1):27−66.
9. Piper EB, Bachman C. The prevention of fetal injuries in breech delivery. *JAMA.* 1929;92(3):217−221.
10. Huber CP, Gynecology. Dührssen's incisions. *Am J Obstet Gynecol.* 1939;37(5):824−834.
11. Burns JW. Breech: A Method of dealing with the Aftercoming Head. *Int J Obstet Gynaecol.* 1934;41(6):923−929.

Vaginal Breech Delivery Simulation

MATERIALS NEEDED
- Model of pelvis
- Fetal manikin
- Piper forceps

KEY PERSONNEL
- Attending obstetrician
- Neonatologist
- Nurse
- Resident physician (if available in your institution)

SAMPLE SCENARIO
A 21-year-old G4P3003 at 38 weeks 4 days presents with painful contractions. On exam, she is found to be 8 cm, 100% effaced, and the presenting part is at 0 station. You suspect, and ultrasound confirms a frank breech presentation. Patient states that she does not want a cesarean delivery.

DEBRIEFING AND DOCUMENTATION
- Type of breech
- Indication for vaginal birth
- Informed consent conversation
- Assessment of maternal pelvis
- Fetal heart rate and contractions
- Progress in labor, including length of second stage
- Maneuvers or manipulations required
- Duration between crowning and complete delivery of the fetus
- If forceps used—number of attempts, ease of application, and duration of traction
- Description of maternal and/or neonatal injuries

Simulation Checklist

		Time	Comments
Initial response	Recognized breech presentation		
	Ultrasound performed for A) Type of breech B) Estimated fetal weight C) Head flexion		
	Assembled appropriate help		
	Obtained consent from patient for vaginal delivery		
	Assembled necessary equipment		
Management	Ensured proper anesthesia		
	Allowed fetus to descend spontaneously until scapulae visible		
	Freed loop of cord to reduce cord tension		
	Rotated fetus to sacrum anterior position		
	Delivered legs with Pinard's maneuver		
	Delivered arms with Løvset's maneuver		
	Delivered head with Mauriceau-Smellie-Veit maneuver or Piper forceps		
Documentation	Timing of events		
	Persons present		
Communication	Kept patient and partner informed		
	Call-out		
	Directed communication		
	Closed-loop communication		

Technical Skills	Non-Technical Skills
List criteria for vaginal breech delivery	Communicate with team members
Describe labor management for vaginal breech delivery	Assess appropriateness of patient for vaginal breech delivery
Demonstrate delivery maneuvers for breech fetus	Communicate with patient

Let's debrief. . .

Technical and nontechnical skills for vaginal breech delivery.

CHAPTER 12

Breech Extraction of a Second Twin

LEARNING OBJECTIVES

- Identify indication for breech extraction.
- Describe technique for breech extraction.
- Identify potential difficulties encountered during breech extraction

Breech extraction has been performed for a long time with different results among the operators.[1-3] It is usually used to describe the delivery of the second twin with vertex-breech presentations. Breech extraction is preferred over passive delivery of a breech second twin.[4] It is reasonable to avoid the procedure when the weight of the second twin is either <1500 or >4000 g, and when the second twin is much larger than the first twin.[5] Of course, the experience of the operator is paramount to its success. Following the delivery of the first twin, the following steps are used for the breech delivery of the second twin:

- With ultrasound assess (a) the heart rate and (b) the presentation of the second twin
- Inform the patient on the steps for the delivery of the twin
- Do not rupture the membranes yet
- Place a hand in vagina and grasp the feet as in Fig 12.1 (it is important to differentiate between hands and feet)
- Pull the feet through the vagina and vulva. There will be fetal resistance that is proportional to fetal weight (Fig. 12.2)
- Continue with gentle extraction and deliver legs, thighs, and buttocks (Fig. 12.3)
- Continue with the delivery as reported in Figs. 11.6–11.7

It is preferable that the membranes are ruptured following the delivery of the lower extremities. However, if they rupture earlier, that is not a problem.

Usually, the back of the fetus rotates anteriorly.

If the back rotates posteriorly, following delivery of the upper extremities, the fetus is elevated toward the maternal abdomen with one hand; two fingers of the other hand are placed around the neck and above the shoulders (Prague maneuver) and the fetus is delivered, as is detailed in Fig. 12.4.

WHAT CAN GO WRONG THAT OUGHT TO BE CORRECTED?

Nuchal Arm

One or both arms may be found around the back of the neck.

In case of only one nuchal arm, the following maneuvers are usually applied (Figs. 12.5-12.7):

- Rotate the back of the fetus toward the same side of the nuchal arm
- Introduce three fingers in the vagina. Place the thumb at the axilla level and the other two fingers

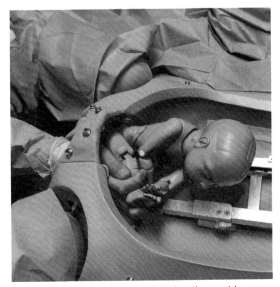

FIG. 12.1 To begin a breech extraction, the provider grasps the baby's feet.

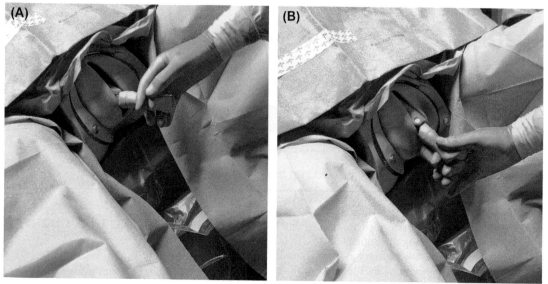

FIG. 12.2 **(A)** One or **(B)** both of the baby's feet are grasped with the provider's hand and pulled through the vagina.

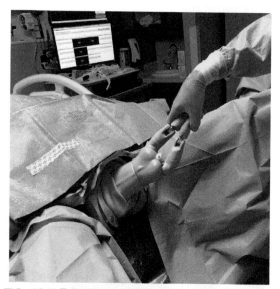

FIG. 12.3 Following the delivery of the baby's torso, the remainder of the breech extraction continues according to the instructions for breech delivery described in the previous chapter.

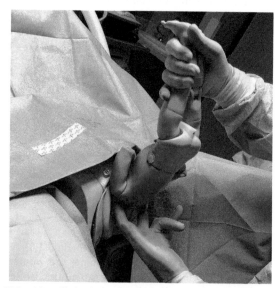

FIG. 12.4 If the baby is delivered with the spine facing down, the baby is elevated toward the mother's abdomen with the provider's right hand. The left hand is used to aid flexion of the head (Prague manuever).

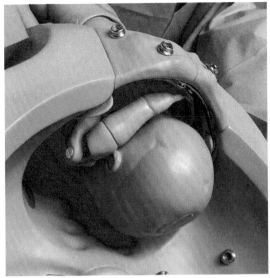

FIG. 12.5 A nuchal arm can obstruct breech delivery.

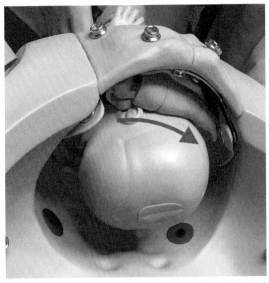

FIG. 12.6 The first step in resolving a nuchal arm is to rotate the baby toward the nuchal arm.

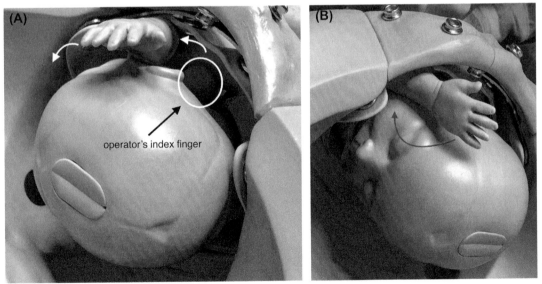

FIG. 12.7 Finally to resolve a nuchal arm, **(A)** introduce three fingers in vagina. Place the thumb at the axilla level and the other two fingers anteriorly to the arm and **(B)** draw the arm anteriorly across the body.

anteriorly to the arm and draw the arm anteriorly across the body.
- If there are bilateral nuchal arm correct one side and then the second side.

Fetal Head Entrapment

- If the cervix constricts the fetal head, the first step is administration of nitroglycerine IV (100 micrograms)[6]
- If this is not successful, Dührsenn incisions become necessary
- If despite the Dührsenn incisions, the head is not delivered, the Zavanelli maneuver is the next step

HOW MUCH TIME DOES THE OBSTETRICIAN HAVE FROM THE TIME THE TRUNK IS DELIVERED TO THE DELIVERY OF THE HEAD?

There is not much information on this topic. Anecdotally, one of my teachers once told me that he had a difficult situation in a case of a breech delivery and finally he was able to deliver the baby's head in 12 minutes. The infant did well.

REFERENCES

1. Davis CH. Version and breech extraction. *Postgrad Med.* 1949;5(5):368–374.
2. Goethals TR. Breech extraction. *Clin Obstet Gynecol.* 1958; 1(4):908–916.
3. Lindsay LM. Breech extraction as a cause of cord laceration and paraplegia. *Can Med Assoc J.* 1926;16(10): 1228–1230.
4. Cruikshank DP. Intrapartum management of twin gestations. *Obstet Gynecol.* 2007;109(5):1167–1176.
5. Gocke SE, et al. Management of the nonvertex second twin: primary cesarean section, external version, or primary breech extraction. *Am J Obstet Gynecol.* 1989;161(1): 111–114.
6. Dofour P, Vinatier D, Puech F. The use of intravenous nitroglycerin for cervico-uterine relaxation: a review of the literature. *Arch Gynecol Obest.* 1997;261:1–7.

Breech Extraction Simulation

MATERIALS NEEDED
- Model of pelvis
- Fetal manikin
- Piper forceps
- Ultrasound

KEY PERSONNEL
- Anesthesiologist
- Attending obstetrician
- Neonatologist
- Nurse
- Resident physician (if available in your institution)

SAMPLE SCENARIO

A 23-year-old G3P2002 at 37 weeks 4 days with dichorionic twin gestation presents in active labor. Initial sonogram shows Baby A in vertex presentation and Baby B in complete breech presentation. The patient is motivated for a vaginal delivery. After an uncomplicated delivery of Baby A, describe your management of Baby B.

DEBRIEFING AND DOCUMENTATION
- Informed consent conversation
- Assessment of fetal heart rate
- Assessment of fetal position
- Maneuvers or manipulations required
- Interval between delivery of Baby A and Baby B
- If forceps used—number of attempts, ease of application, and duration of traction
- Description of maternal and/or neonatal injuries

Simulation Checklist

		Time	Comments
Initial response	Ultrasound performed for fetal heart rate and presentation		
	Breech presentation identified		
Management	Feet identified and grasped		
	Feet drawn through the vagina		
	Freed loop of cord to reduce cord tension		
	Rotated fetus to sacrum anterior position		
	Complete the extraction if possible		
	Delivered arms with LøvseT's maneuver, as necessary		
	Delivered head with Mauriceau– Smellie–Veit maneuver or Piper forceps, as necessary		
Documentation	Timing of events		
	Persons present		
Communication	Kept patient and partner informed		
	Directed communication		
	Closed-loop communication		

Technical Skills	Non-Technical Skills
Ultrasound identification of fetal position	Communication with team members
Grasping of fetal legs	Informed consent with patient
Resolution of nuchal arm	Task management
Delivery of entrapped head	Teamwork

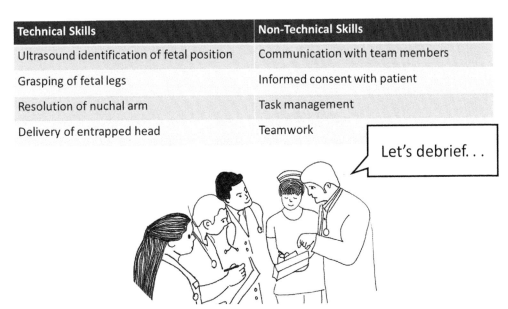

Let's debrief. . .

Technical and nontechnical skills for breech extraction.

Umbilical Cord Prolapse

Umbilical cord prolapse is a condition in which the umbilical cord presents ahead of the presenting part of the fetus. The umbilical cord will typically protrude into the cervix, vagina, or outside of the body. Cord prolapse is considered an obstetric emergency because of the risk of complications including cord compression, umbilical artery vasospasm, and umbilical vein obstruction, all of which lead to the risk of fetal oxygenation compromise.

RISK FACTORS[1,2]

- Unengaged presenting part due to maternal or fetal factors
- Fetal malpresentation
  - Footling breech—15% risk of cord prolapse
  - Complete breech—5% risk of cord prolapse
  - Frank breech—0.5% risk of cord prolapse (which is equivalent to cephalic)
- Prematurity
- Low birth weight
- Second twin
- Fetal anomalies
- Polyhydramnios
- Long umbilical cord
- Low lying placenta
- Maternal pelvic deformities
- Uterine tumors or malformations
- Multiparity
- Artificial rupture of membranes with an unengaged presenting part
- Cervical ripening with a balloon catheter
- Induction of labor
- Application of an internal scalp electrode
- Insertion of an intrauterine pressure catheter
- Manual rotation of the fetal head

- Amnioinfusion
- External cephalic version
- Internal podalic version
- Application of forceps or vacuum

PREVENTION[2-4]

- Avoid unnecessary obstetric interventions and perform necessary interventions with care
- Awareness of patients at high risk is key to enable prompt diagnosis and management if prolapse occurs
- Patient with antepartum diagnosis of funic presentation should be followed closely until time of delivery. Funic presentation will resolve in many patients with the onset of labor

DIAGNOSIS[5,6]

- Most commonly presents with an abrupt onset of sustained, severe fetal bradycardia or repetitive, severe variable decelerations in a patient with previous Category I tracing
- Pulsating umbilical cord may be palpated on cervical examination
- Patient may report seeing or feeling an overt cord prolapse
- Diagnosis is made based on visualization or palpation of the umbilical cord ahead of the presenting fetal part

MANAGEMENT[5-7] (FIG. 13.1)

- CALL FOR HELP!! Necessary personnel include the following:
  - An experienced care provider

Safety Training for Obstetric Emergencies. https://doi.org/10.1016/B978-0-323-69672-2.00013-8

(A)

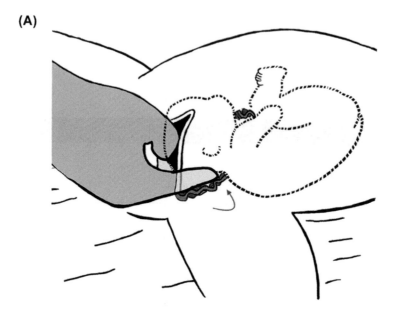

(B)

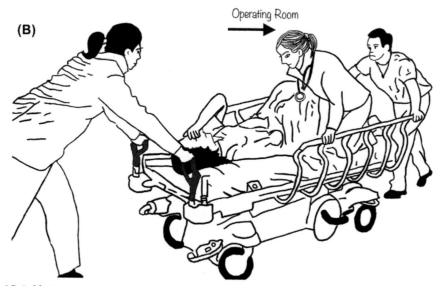

FIG. 13.1 Management of cord prolapse. **(A)** The goal is to reduce cord compression while **(B)** moving toward emergent cesarean section. An assistant elevates the presenting part while the woman is placed in Trendelenburg or knee-chest position.

- Two labor and delivery nurses
- A neonatologist
- An anesthesiologist
- Operating room staff
- State clearly "There is a cord prolapse."
- Prepare for emergency cesarean delivery
- Initiate maneuvers for intrauterine resuscitation
  - **Manual elevation of the presenting fetal part**—elevate the presenting fetal part with care to alleviate umbilical cord compression as preparations are made for cesarean delivery. Avoid further cord compression or cord manipulation, which can trigger vasospasm
  - **Place the patient in Trendelenburg or knee-chest position**
  - **Retrofill the bladder**—fill the bladder with 500—700 mL of saline via a catheter to lift the presenting part and alleviate compression
  - **Administer a tocolytic**
- Continuously monitor fetal heart rate—allows assessment of effective intrauterine resuscitation
- Perform an emergent cesarean delivery. If the provider is delivering intrauterine resuscitation, he or she should continue elevation of the presenting fetal part until just before delivery of the presenting part through the uterine incision. Therefore, it is necessary for a second provider to perform the cesarean delivery

- Type of anesthesia depends on the adequacy of preexisting anesthesia and fetal status

REFERENCES

1. Hasegawa J, et al. The use of balloons for uterine cervical ripening is associated with an increased risk of umbilical cord prolapse: population based questionnaire survey in Japan. *BMC Pregnancy Childbirth*. 2015;15:4.
2. Behbehani S, Patenaude V, Abenhaim HA. Maternal risk factors and outcomes of umbilical cord prolapse: a population-based study. *J Obstet Gynaecol Can*. 2016;38(1):23—28.
3. Holbrook BD, Phelan ST. Umbilical cord prolapse. *Obstet Gynecol Clin N Am*. 2013;40(1):1—14.
4. Struble J, Mytopher K. Overt cord prolapse diagnosed at ultrasound. *J Obstet Gynaecol Can*. 2018;40(3):271.
5. Maher MD, Heavey E. When the cord comes first: umbilical cord prolapse. *Nursing*. 2015;45(7):53—56.
6. Rajakumar C, et al. Umbilical cord prolapse in a labouring patient: a multidisciplinary and interprofessional simulation scenario. *Cureus*. 2017;9(9):e1692.
7. Copson S, et al. The effect of a multidisciplinary obstetric emergency team training program, the in Time course, on diagnosis to delivery interval following umbilical cord prolapse — a retrospective cohort study. *Aust N Z J Obstet Gynaecol*. 2017;57(3):327—333.

Umbilical Cord Prolapse Simulation

MATERIALS NEEDED
- Manikin-should be as realistic as your budget and supplies allow. At the very least, a manikin allows one to check for cord prolapse and perform maneuvers to reduce cord compression

KEY PERSONNEL
- Anesthesiologist
- Attending obstetrician
- Neonatologist
- Operating room staff
- Resident physician (if available in your institution)
- Two nurses

SAMPLE SCENARIO
Angela is a 24-year-old G3P0202 at 32 weeks gestation who was admitted 2 days ago with preterm prelabor rupture of membranes. She is being observed on the floor when she calls out that she "feels something between her legs." Her nurse reports to her room and notes a loop of umbilical cord protruding from her vagina.

DEBRIEFING
- Risk factors for cord prolapse
- Time cord prolapsed recognized, how diagnosis was made
- Time emergency response protocol initiated
- Time in OR
- Time of delivery
- Interventions implemented to decrease cord compression
- Did continuous fetal heart rate monitoring take place?
- Type of anesthesia used
- Description of maternal and neonatal condition
  - Fetal weight
  - Cord gas
  - APGAR scores
  - Resuscitation
- Communication with patient and family

Simulation Checklist

		Time	Comments
Initial response	Recognized cord prolapse		
	Called for help		
	Initiated protocol for emergency cesarean delivery		
	Communicated clearly "we have a prolapsed cord."		
Management	Performed immediate vaginal exam		
	Elevated presenting part		
	Minimized manipulation of the cord		
	Repositioned mother to reduce cord compression (knee-chest or Trendelenburg)		
	Continuous fetal monitoring		
	Started IV		
	Prepared for neonatal resuscitation		
Documentation	Timing of events		
	Persons present		
Communication	Kept patient and partner informed		
	Call-out		
	Directed communication		
	Closed-loop communication		

Technical Skills	Non-Technical Skills
List risk factors for umbilical cord prolapse	Use call-out communication
Demonstrate technique for elevation of presenting fetal part	Assign team roles
Perform cesarean delivery	Communicate with patient
Resuscitate neonate	Debrief with team

Let's debrief. . .

Technical and nontechnical skills for umbilical cord prolapse.

Antepartum Hemorrhage

Antepartum hemorrhage is defined as any bleeding from the genital tract after the 20th week of pregnancy and before the onset of labor. Antepartum hemorrhage complicates 2%–5% of all pregnancies[1]. It is associated with increased rates of perinatal morbidity and mortality and contributes significantly to health-care costs.

CAUSES OF ANTEPARTUM HEMORRHAGE[1]

- Placenta previa
- Placental abruption
- Uterine rupture
- Vasa previa
- Cervical lesions (such as polyps, ectropion, or malignancy)
- Infection
- Trauma
- Unknownk

COMPLICATIONS[2-3]

- Maternal hypovolemic shock
- Premature birth

TYPES OF ANTEPARTUM HEMORRHAGE

Placental Abruption (Fig. 14.1)

Placental abruption, or abruptio placentae, occurs when the placenta separates from the lining of the uterus prior to delivery. Patients typically present with bleeding in setting of abdominal pain. There are two types of placental abruption:

- **Revealed placental abruption** causes overt vaginal bleeding

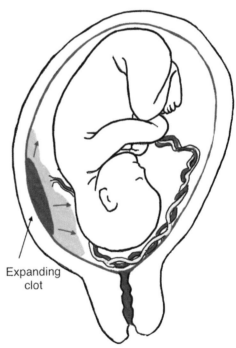

FIG. 14.1 Placental abruption. This occurs when the placenta separates from the uterine wall. It typically presents with painful vaginal bleeding.

- **Concealed placental abruption** occurs when there is no vaginal bleeding because the blood gets trapped inside the uterus behind the placenta

Placenta Previa[4-5]

Placenta previa is abnormal implantation of the placenta over the internal cervical os. The classification

(A)

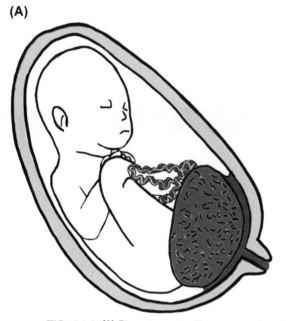

(B)

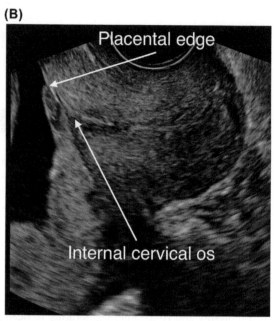

FIG. 14.2 **(A)** Placenta previa. This occurs when the placenta overlies the internal cervical os. It typically presents with painless vaginal bleeding. **(B)** Ultrasound image of placenta previa, with lower placental edge, completely covering internal cervical os.

of placenta previa has recently been simplified as follows:

- **Placenta previa** is defined when the placental overlies the internal cervical os (Fig. 14.2)

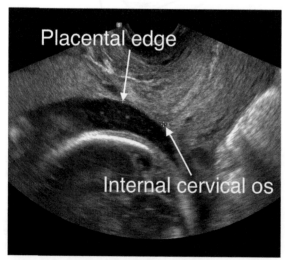

FIG. 14.3 Ultrasound image of "low lying placenta" (lower placental edge within 2cm of internal cervical os).

- **Low-lying placenta** is defined when the placental edge is within 2 cm of but not covering the internal cervical os (Fig. 14.3)

DIAGNOSIS AND EVALUATION

- History
  - Expected due date/gestational age
  - Timing and amount of blood loss (number of pads used, estimation of blood staining on each pad)
  - Associated features (abdominal pain, contractions)
  - Provoking factors (trauma, sexual intercourse)
  - Fetal movements since the bleeding started
  - Previous episodes of bleeding in current pregnancy
  - Ultrasounds performed earlier in pregnancy, particularly noting placental site recorded on a 20-week (or later) scan

Ultrasound

- Ultrasound is used to assess for placental and vascular abnormalities. This should be performed *before* vaginal examination
- An ultrasound scan is **not** the investigation of choice to diagnose a placental abruption; placental

abruption is diagnosed clinically based on painful contractions and vaginal bleeding

Physical Exam

- Abdominal palpation for uterine tenderness and symphysis-fundal height, fetal lie and presentation
- Vaginal/cervical examination is contraindicated in patients who present with painless third-trimester vaginal bleeding until a placenta previa can be ruled out by ultrasound. A digital cervical exam in a patient with a placenta previa can cause catastrophic hemorrhage. After placenta previa is ruled out, a speculum exam can help identify the source of the bleeding

Laboratory Tests

- Blood type and antibody screen
- CBC
- Kleihauer–Betke test
- APTT, PT, fibrin degradation products
- Note blood loss (amount, consistency, and color)
- Assess fetal well-being

MANAGEMENT

Resuscitation

- Remember—changes in maternal vitals are a late sign!
- Record the patient's pulse, blood pressure, temperature, respiratory rate, and oxygen saturation level
- Important steps for volume replacement:
  - Obtain IV access with one or two 18-gauge or larger bore IV lines
  - Infuse fluids at approximately the rate that blood is being lost. In initial resuscitation, fluid replacement with crystalloid is as effective as with colloid
- Insert an indwelling urinary catheter with urometer and record hourly urine output
- Consider need for blood transfusion

Medications

- The need for analgesia should raise concerns of a moderate/severe placental abruption or that the woman is in labor. Offer analgesia and antiemetic medications if indicated
- Give corticosteroids if gestational age is less than 34 weeks

REFERENCES

1. Ananth CV, Wilcox AJ, Savitz DA. Effect of maternal age and parity on the risk of uteroplacental bleeding disorders in pregnancy. *Obstet Gynecol.* 1996;88(4 Pt 1):511–516.
2. Towers CV, Burkhart AE. Pregnancy outcome after a primary antenatal hemorrhage between 16 and 24 weeks' gestation. *SO Am J Obstet Gynecol.* 2008;198(6):684.e1. Epub 2008 Apr 25.
3. Bhandari S, Raja EA, Shetty A, Bhattacharya S. Maternal and perinatal consequences of antepartum haemorrhage of unknown origin.
4. Reddy UM, et al. Fetal imaging: executive summary of a joint Eunice Kennedy Shriver National Institute of Child Health and Human Development, Society for maternal-fetal medicine, American Institute of ultrasound in medicine, American College of obstetricians and Gynecologists, American College of Radiology, Society for Pediatric Radiology, and Society of Radiologists in ultrasound fetal Imaging workshop. *Obstet Gynecol.* 2014; 123(5):1070–1082.
5. Daskalakis G, et al. Impact of placenta previa on obstetric outcome. *Int J Gynaecol Obstet.* 2011;114(3):238–241.

Antepartum Hemorrhage Simulation

MATERIALS NEEDED
- Manikin or volunteer to act as standardized patient

KEY PERSONNEL
- Anesthesiologist
- Attending obstetrician
- Neonatologist
- Operating room staff
- Resident physician (if available in your institution)
- Two nurses

SAMPLE SCENARIO
Maria is a 28-year-old G3P2002 at 32 weeks gestation by stated LMP who presents to triage complaining of vaginal bleeding that began after intercourse. Patient has not had any prenatal care yet this pregnancy. On exam, BP 110/45, P 99, RR 14, SpO$_2$ 97%. Her pants and underwear are saturated with blood and you can note active bleeding coming from the vagina.

DEBRIEFING
- Diagnosis
- Fluid input and output
- Events and interventions performed
- Blood transfused
- Maternal vital signs
- Fetal status

Simulation Checklist

		Time	Comments
Recognize	Recognized abnormal fetal heart rate pattern		
	Recognized constant abdominal pain despite epidural		
	Performed abdominal assessment		
	Performed vaginal assessment		
	Recognized risk factors in clinical history		
	Recognized cause of antepartum hemorrhage		
Call for help	Summoned appropriate help urgently		
	Called for experienced help (including neonatologist once decision made to expedite delivery)		
	Repositioned woman in left-lateral position		
Management	Administered high flow O_2 via nonrebreather		
	Established IV access		
	Estimated blood loss		
	Checked CBC, PT/INR, PTT		
	Planned for emergent cesarean delivery		
	Transferred patient to the operating room		
	Administered additional medications as ordered		
	Used appropriate anesthesia		
	Ordered type and Cross for two units		
Fluids	Total IV fluid bolus LR 1000 mL/h		
	Blood transfusion		
Monitoring	Blood pressure/respiratory rate/O_2 saturation		
	Urinary output		
	Electronic fetal monitoring (after mother stabilized) until birth		
Documentation	Timing of events		
	Medications administered		
	Persons present		
Communication	Call-out		
	Directed communication		
	Closed-loop communication		

Technical Skills	Non-Technical Skills
List causes of antepartum hemorrhage	Determine urgency of situation
Recognize placenta previa on ultrasound	Assign team roles
Obtain IV access	Use directed communication
Apply fetal monitors	Communicate with patient

Let's debrief. . .

Technical and nontechnical skills for antepartum hemorrhage.

Vasa Previa

The term vasa previa refers to fetal blood vessels present in the membranes covering or within 2 cm of the internal cervical os[1]. These vessels are not protected by Wharton's jelly and are at risk for rupture upon spontaneous or artificial rupture of the membranes. Their presence can be a result of either velamentous cord insertion or a succenturiate lobe. If fetal bleeding occurs, fetal exsanguination can occur within minutes. These vessels are also at risk of compression from the presenting part, and compression can lead to asphyxia (Fig. 15.1).

RISK FACTORS[2-5]

- Use of assisted reproductive technologies
- Second-trimester low-lying placenta/placenta previa (even if resolved)
- Bilobed or succenturiate lobe placentas in the lower uterine segment
- Velamentous cord insertion
- Multiple gestations

DIAGNOSIS[6-9]

Perinatal mortality is <3% when it is diagnosed antenatally. Mortality rises to nearly 60% when vasa previa is diagnosed intrapartum or postpartum[5]

Ultrasound findings

- Linear sonolucent area crossing over the internal os. Color Doppler flow reveals arterial or venous waveforms (Fig. 15.2)
- The placenta is often low-lying, bilobed, or succenturiate

Physical exam findings

- Very rarely, pulsating vessels in the membranes overlying the cervical os can be palpated

Clinical findings

- A clinical diagnosis should be suspected when there is vaginal bleeding upon rupture of the membranes with fetal heart rate abnormalities, especially a sinusoidal pattern or bradycardia

Laboratory testing

- The Apt test has been described to differentiate fetal versus maternal bleeding. However, the emergent nature of bleeding vasa previa precludes the clinical utility of this test.

DIFFERENTIAL DIAGNOSIS[10]

- Funic presentation: A loop of umbilical cord overlying the cervical os
- Cervico—uterine vessels[10]
- Amniotic band or chorioamniotic separation

MANAGEMENT[11-14]

Antenatal

- Consider betamethasone between 28 and 32 weeks of gestation due to increased risk of emergent preterm delivery
- Consider hospital admission between 30 and 34 weeks of gestation with NST 2—3 times daily
- Emergency cesarean delivery should be performed promptly if cord compression or early labor is detected, ideally before rupture of membranes

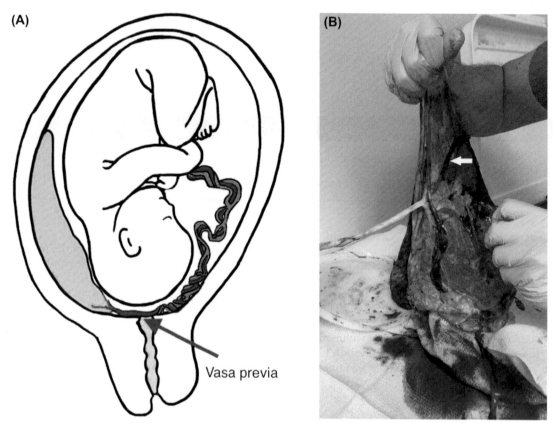

FIG. 15.1 Vasa previa. **(A)** This condition is defined by the fetal blood vessels embedded in the membranes within 2 cm of the internal cervical os. These fetal vessels do not have protective Wharton's jelly. Figure **(B)** shows placenta after delivery. The arrow indicates fetal vessels that were located above cervical os.

Delivery

- Delivery via cesarean delivery is recommended between 34 and 37 weeks of gestation
- Earlier delivery by emergency cesarean delivery is indicated in case of:
  - Labor
  - Rupture of membranes
  - Repetitive variable decelerations
  - Vaginal bleeding with fetal surveillance changes such as fetal tachycardia, sinusoidal heart rate pattern, or evidence of pure fetal blood by Apt test or Kleihauer–Betke assessment[9]
- The hysterotomy should avoid aberrant blood vessels. If a fetal vessel is lacerated during delivery, the cord should be clamped immediately to prevent fetal/neonatal blood loss
- Type O negative blood should be available for emergency transfusion of a severely anemic newborn

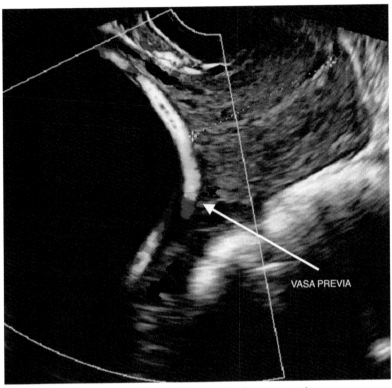

FIG. 15.2 Ultrasound image showing vasa previa.

REFERENCES

1. Oyelese Y, Smulian JC. Placenta previa, placenta accreta, and vasa previa. *Obstet Gynecol.* 2006;107:927–941.
2. Schachter M, Tovbin Y, Arieli S, Friedler S, Ron-El R, Sherman D. In vitro fertilization is a risk factor for vasa previa. *Fertil Steril.* 2002;78:642–643.
3. Bronsteen R, Whitten A, Balasubramanian M, et al. Vasa previa: clinical presentations, out- comes, and implications for management. *Obstet Gynecol.* 2013;122:352–357.
4. Baulies S, Maiz N, Munoz A, Torrents M, Echevarria M, Serra B. Prenatal ultrasound diagnosis of vasa praevia and analysis of risk factors. *Prenat Diagn.* 2007;27:595–599.
5. Oyelese Y, Catanzarite V, Prefumo F, et al. Vasa previa: the impact of prenatal diagnosis on outcomes. *Obstet Gynecol.* 2004;103:937–942.
6. Silver RM. Abnormal placentation: placenta previa, vasa previa, and placenta accreta. *Obstet Gynecol.* 2015;126(3):654–668.
7. Lee W, Lee VL, Kirk JS, Sloan CT, Smith RS, Comstock CH. Vasa previa: prenatal diagnosis, natural evolution, and clinical outcome. *Obstet Gynecol.* 2000;95(4):572–576.
8. Rebarber A, Dolin C, Fox NS, Klauser CK, Saltzman DH, Roman AS. Natural history of vasa previa across gestation using a screening protocol. *J Ultrasound Med.* 2014;33(1):141–147.
9. Odunsi K, Bullough CH, Henzel J, Polanska A. Evaluation of chemical tests for fetal bleeding from vasa previa. *Int J Gynaecol Obstet.* 1996;55(3):207–212.
10. Swank ML, Garite TJ, Maurel K, Das A, Perlow JH, Combs CA, Fishman S, Vanderhoeven J, Nageotte M, Bush M, Lewis D. Obstetrix Collaborative Research Network. *Am J Obstet Gynecol.* 2016;215(2):223. e1–6.
11. Gagnon R, Morin L, Bly S, et al. SOGC clinical practice guideline: guidelines for the management of vasa previa. *Int J Gynaecol Obstet.* 2010;108:85–89.
12. Hasegawa J, Arakaki T, Ichizuka K. Sekizawa. Management of vasa previa during pregnancy. *J Perinat Med.* 2015;43(6):783–784.
13. Society of Maternal-Fetal Publications C, Sinkey RG, Odibo AO, Dashe JS. #37: diagnosis and management of vasa previa. *Am J Obstet Gynecol.* 2015;213(5):615–619.
14. Gomes A, Rezende J, Vogt MF, Zaconeta A. Vasa previa: a cautious approach at caesarean section. *J Obstet Gynaecol Can.* 2017;39(4):203–204.

Vasa Previa Simulation

MATERIALS NEEDED
- Manikin or volunteer to act as standardized patient

KEY PERSONNEL
- Anesthesiologist
- Attending obstetrician
- Neonatologist
- Operating room staff
- Resident physician (if available in your institution)
- Two nurses

SAMPLE SCENARIO

A 26-year-old presents with painful contractions at 35 weeks gestation. Her pregnancy has been uncomplicated other than a low-lying placenta diagnosed at her anatomic survey. On transabdominal sonogram you do not appreciate a low-lying placenta. Her cervix is closed. She is being observed on labor and delivery for contractions when she calls out that she is bleeding. Her fetal heart rate monitor shows an abrupt deceleration to 70 beats per minute.

DEBRIEFING AND DOCUMENTATION
- When and how was diagnosis made
- Indication, urgency of delivery
- Description of maternal and/or neonatal injuries
- Communication with patient and family

Simulation Checklist

		Time	Comments
Recognize	Recognized abnormal fetal heart rate pattern		
	Recognized risk factors in clinical history		
	Recognized cause of antepartum hemorrhage		
Call for help	Summoned appropriate help urgently		
	Called for experienced help (including neonatologist once decision made to expedite delivery)		
	Prepared for emergency cesarean		
Management	Transferred patient to the operating room		
	Clamped cord immediately		
	O Negative blood available for neonatal transfusion		
	Used appropriate anesthesia		
Documentation	Timing of events		
	Persons present		
Communication	Call-out		
	Directed communication		
	Closed-loop communication		

Technical Skills	Non-Technical Skills
Define vasa previa	Recognize emergent nature of bleeding vasa previa
Recognize vasa previa on ultrasound	Assign team roles
Perform cesarean delivery	Communicate with patient

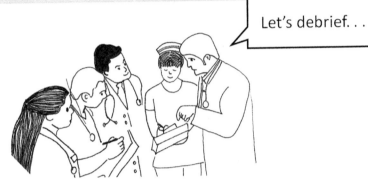

Let's debrief. . .

Technical and nontechnical skills for vasa previa.

CHAPTER 16

Uterine Rupture

LEARNING OBJECTIVES

- List risk factors for uterine rupture.
- Recognize signs of uterine rupture.
- Describe management of uterine rupture.

Uterine rupture, also known as uterine dehiscence, refers to the total or partial disruption of the uterine layers (Fig. 16.1).[1] It is a life-threatening emergency for both the mother and fetus. Most commonly uterine rupture occurs in the context of a "scarred uterus."[2] A "scarred uterus" includes one with any previous uterine surgery, including prior cesarean delivery or myomectomy, especially if the contractile portion of the uterus has been entered.

In high resource countries, uterine rupture is mainly related with trial of labor after cesarean section (TOLAC). In low resource countries, uterine rupture is associated with "obstructed labor."[3]

RISK FACTORS[1-11]

- Prior uterine rupture
- History of classical cesarean

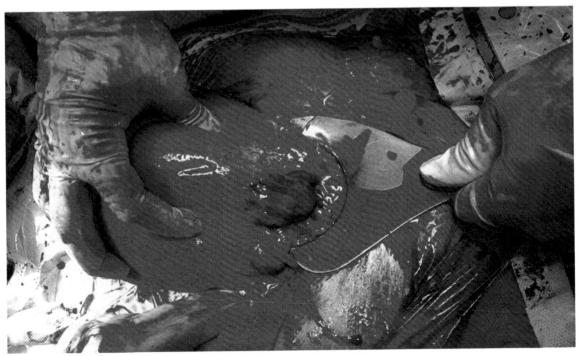

FIG. 16.1 Photograph of uterine rupture.

Safety Training for Obstetric Emergencies. https://doi.org/10.1016/B978-0-323-69672-2.00016-3

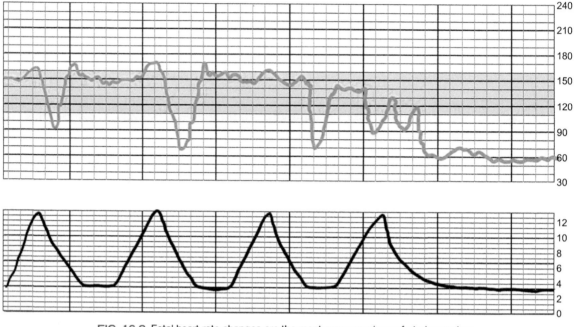

FIG. 16.2 Fetal heart rate changes are the most common signs of uterine rupture.

- Prior myometrial surgery
- Exposure to uterotonics
- Labor
- Multiparity
- Advanced maternal age
- Abnormal placentation
- Short interpregnancy interval
- Macrosomia

A prior vaginal delivery decreases the risk of uterine rupture, either before or after a prior cesarean section.

Unfortunately, there are no accurate and clinically useful predictors of uterine rupture; consequently, a high index of suspicion is needed. Whenever TOLAC is attempted, continuous fetal monitoring is recommended.

INTRAPARTUM SIGNS AND SYMPTOMS[12-15]

- Fetal heart rate abnormalities: This is the most common sign of uterine rupture although no specific pattern is pathognomonic of rupture. Fetal bradycardia is the most common abnormality (Fig. 16.2)
- Sudden onset or worsening abdominal pain; regional anesthesia may mask or attenuate this symptom
- Vaginal bleeding
- Loss of fetal station

- Hematuria
- Hemodynamic changes, secondary to acute blood loss from intraperitoneal hemorrhage
- Change of contractions pattern

POSTPARTUM SIGN AND SYMPTOMS

- Persistent pain
- Persistent vaginal bleeding
- Hematuria
- Hemodynamic changes, secondary to acute blood loss from intraperitoneal hemorrhage

MANAGEMENT

IMMEDIATE DELIVERY is essential.

Simultaneous aggressive fluid and blood products resuscitation should be undertaken.

The choice of general versus regional anesthesia should be balanced against the condition of the fetus and the mother. General anesthesia is the fastest route. Some practitioners offer early regional anesthesia in patients undergoing TOLAC, in case of an emergency.

After emergent delivery is undertaken or in case of postdelivery emergency laparotomy, the goal is to repair the uterine defect, obtain hemostasis, treat complications, and/or repair additional internal organ injuries.

The decision of uterine repair versus hysterectomy is made taking into account several factors. These include the extent of the damage, bleeding control, patient's hemodynamic condition, and patient's reproductive desires.

REFERENCES

1. American College of, O. and Gynecologists. ACOG Practice bulletin no. 115: vaginal birth after previous cesarean delivery. *Obstet Gynecol.* 2010;116(2 Pt 1):450–463.
2. Guise JM, et al. Vaginal birth after cesarean: new insights. *Evid Rep Technol Assess (Full Rep).* 2010;(191):1–397.
3. Hofmeyr GJ, Say L, Gulmezoglu AM. WHO systematic review of maternal mortality and morbidity: the prevalence of uterine rupture. *BJOG.* 2005;112(9):1221–1228.
4. Usta IM, et al. Pregnancy outcome in patients with previous uterine rupture. *Acta Obstet Gynecol Scand.* 2007; 86(2):172–176.
5. Landon MB, et al. Maternal and perinatal outcomes associated with a trial of labor after prior cesarean delivery. *N Engl J Med.* 2004;351(25):2581–2589.
6. Landon MB, Lynch CD. Optimal timing and mode of delivery after cesarean with previous classical incision or myomectomy: a review of the data. *Semin Perinatol.* 2011;35(5):257–261.
7. Lydon-Rochelle M, et al. Risk of uterine rupture during labor among women with a prior cesarean delivery. *N Engl J Med.* 2001;345(1):3–8.
8. Gibbins KJ, et al. Maternal and fetal morbidity associated with uterine rupture of the unscarred uterus. *Am J Obstet Gynecol.* 2015;213(3):382 e1–6.
9. LeMaire WJ, et al. Placenta percreta with spontaneous rupture of an unscarred uterus in the second trimester. *Obstet Gynecol.* 2001;98(5 Pt 2):927–929.
10. Al-Zirqi I, Daltveit AK, Forsén L, Stray-Pedersen B, Vangen S. Risk factors for complete uterine rupture. *Am J Obstet Gynecol.* 2017;216(2):165.e1–165.e8.
11. Ayres AW, Johnson TR, Hayashi R. Characteristics of fetal heart rate tracings prior to uterine rupture. *Int J Gynaecol Obstet.* 2001;74(3):235–240.
12. Guiliano M, et al. Signs, symptoms and complications of complete and partial uterine ruptures during pregnancy and delivery. *Eur J Obstet Gynecol Reprod Biol.* 2014;179: 130–134.
13. Landon MB, Spong CY, Thom E, et al. National Institute of Child Health and Human Development Maternal-Fetal Medicine Units Network. Risk of uterine rupture with a trial of labor in women with multiple and single prior cesarean delivery. *Obstet Gynecol.* 2006;108(1): 12–20.
14. Markou GA, Muray JM, Poncelet C. Risk factors and symptoms associated with maternal and neonatal complications in women with uterine rupture. A 16 years multicentric experience. *Eur J Obstet Gynecol Reprod Biol.* 2017;217:126–130.
15. Craver Pryor E, et al. Intrapartum predictors of uterine rupture. *Am J Perinatol.* 2007;24(5):317–321.

Uterine Rupture Simulation

MATERIALS NEEDED
- Manikin or volunteer to act as standardized patient

KEY PERSONNEL
- Anesthesiologist
- Attending obstetrician
- Neonatologist
- Resident physician (if available in your institution)
- Two nurses

SAMPLE SCENARIO
Ji-Young is a 26-year-old G2P1 at 38 weeks 4 days gestation presented in labor. She has a history of one previous cesarean delivery and is highly motivated for vaginal delivery. Her initial exam is 5 cm dilated, 50% effaced, and −1 station. She is admitted and is preparing for an epidural when she experiences sudden worsening of pain. The fetal heart rate tracing shows a prolonged deceleration to 60 beats per minute.

DEBRIEFING AND DOCUMENTATION
- Risk factors for uterine rupture
- Time uterine rupture recognized, how diagnosis was made
- Time emergency response protocol initiated
- Time in OR
- Time of delivery
- Interventions implemented while preparations were done for emergency delivery
- Review of continuous fetal heart rate monitoring, did it take place?
- Type of anesthesia used
- Surgical technique employed to manage the rupture
- Description of maternal and neonatal condition.
  - Fetal weight
  - Cord gas
  - APGAR scores
  - Resuscitation
- Communication with patient and family

Simulation Checklist		Time	Comments
Recognize	Recognized abnormal fetal heart rate pattern		
	Recognized risk factors in clinical history		
	Recognized cause of antepartum or postpartum hemorrhage		
Call for help	Summoned appropriate help urgently		
	Called for experienced help (including neonatologist, anesthesiologist, additional surgeons once decision made to expedite delivery)		
	Prepared for emergency cesarean		
Management	Transferred patient to the operating room		
	Immediate laparotomy		
	Immediate delivery		
	Simultaneous fluid and blood product resuscitation while preparing for the operating room		
	Use of appropriate anesthesia		
Documentation	Timing of events		
	Persons present		
Communication	Call-out		
	Directed communication		
	Closed-loop communication		

Technical Skills	Non-Technical Skills
Recognition of worrisome changes in fetal heart rate tracing	Communication with patient regarding risks and benefits of trial of labor after cesarean
Performance of cesarean delivery	Documentation of patient's likelihood of successful trial of labor
Timely delivery of anesthesia for cesarean	Task management
Repair of uterine rupture	Teamwork

Let's debrief. . .

Technical and nontechnical skills for management of uterine rupture.

Postpartum Hemorrhage

Postpartum hemorrhage (PPH) is defined as cumulative blood loss greater than or equal to 1000 mL or excessive blood loss leading to development of symptoms (i.e., lightheaded, vertigo, syncope) and signs of hypovolemia (i.e., hypotension, tachycardia, or oliguria)[1]

CLASSIFICATION OF POSTPARTUM HEMORRHAGE

Postpartum hemorrhage affects 5%–15% of women giving birth. PPH can be categorized into one of two categories:
- Early (primary)
  - Occurs within the first 24 hours
  - Etiologies (think the "4 T's"):
    - Uterine atony (80%–90% of cases)
    - Tissue—retained products of conception
    - Trauma—uterine, cervical or vaginal lacerations
    - Thrombin—dilutional or consumptive coagulopathy, coagulation disorders
- Late (secondary)
  - Occurs between 24 hours and sixth week postpartum
  - Most likely to occur from 6 to 14 days postpartum
  - Etiology is usually infection, uterine subinvolution, or retained placental tissue

RISK FACTORS[1-5]

- Overdistended uterus, as caused by polyhydramnios or multiple gestations
- Macrosomia
- Prolonged labor
- Extended third stage of labor
- High parity
- Fibroid uterus or other uterine anomalies
- Placenta previa
- Cesarean delivery
- Episiotomy
- Trauma and lacerations
- Use of forceps or vacuum device
- History of uterine atony or hemorrhage
- Use of general anesthesia

POSTPARTUM ASSESSMENT

- Prompt and accurate identification of the signs and symptoms of postpartum hemorrhage is key
- Typical schedule of evaluation:
  - Every 15 minutes for 1 hour, then
  - Every 30 minutes for 1 hour, then
  - Every hour for 4 hours, then
  - Every 4 hours for first 24 hours, then
  - Every 8 hours until discharge
- Expect a slight increase in lochia with ambulation and breastfeeding

QUANTIFICATION OF BLOOD LOSS[6]

- Quantification of blood loss improves accuracy of estimated blood loss related to PPH
- Accomplished by knowing totaling measurements of blood in collection devices. Commonly used values are shown in Figs. 17.1 and 17.2.

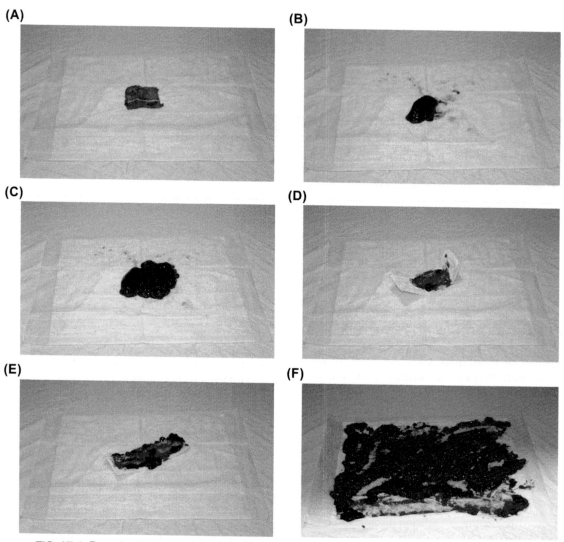

(A) **(B)** **(C)** **(D)** **(E)** **(F)**

FIG. 17.1 Examples of blood loss. **(A)** Soaked 4 × 4 = 5 mL. **(B)** Fist-sized clot = 60 mL. **(C)** Soda can-sized clot = 355 mL. **(D)** Partially soaked peripad = 50 mL. **(E)** Peripad = 70 mL. **(F)** Full, dripping Chux = 800 mL. **(G)** 1/2 saturated lap sponge = 50 mL. **(H)** Full lap sponge = 75 mL. **(I)** Full, dripping lap sponge = 100 mL.

MANAGEMENT OF POSTPARTUM HEMORRHAGE

Active Management of the Third Stage of Labor

- Begin uterotonic drugs after the delivery of the anterior shoulder
- Ensure uterine contractions after delivery of placenta by fundal palpation and bimanual massage if necessary
- Inspect placenta for completeness

Identify the Etiology of the Hemorrhage

- Palpate the abdomen: assess uterine tone
- Inspect the cervix, vagina, vulva, and perianal area for lacerations, hematomas, or uterine inversion
- Perform manual exploration of uterine cavity to remove clots and retained tissue
- Consider coagulopathy. These may include the following:
  - Hemophilia A
  - Von Willebrand's disease

(G) **(H)**

(I)

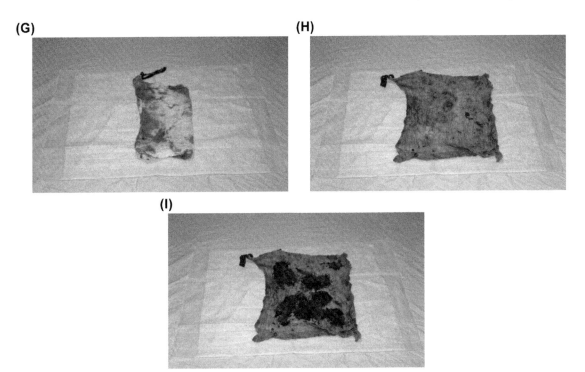

FIG. 17.1 cont'd.

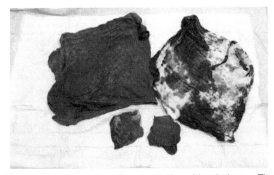

FIG. 17.2 Example of quantitative blood loss. The measured blood loss is 75 mL (full lap) + 50 mL (half lap) + 5 mL (4 × 4) + 5 mL (4 × 4). It is therefore recorded as 135 mL.

- Liver disease
- Therapeutic anticoagulation
- Thrombocytopenia
- Disseminated intravascular coagulation (from preeclampsia, intrauterine fetal demise, severe infection, placental abruption, or amniotic fluid embolism)

Approach to Uterine Atony[1,7]

- **Begin with bimanual fundal massage** (Fig. 17.3)
- **Uterotonic agents** (Table. 17.1)
  - Rapid, continuous infusion of dilute IV Oxytocin (40−80 units in 1L normal saline)
  - Misoprostol (Cytotec, PGE_1) 800−1000 mcg orally, sublingually, vaginally, or rectally
  - Methylergonovine maleate (Methergine) 0.2 mg IM repeated every 2−4 hours as needed up to five doses. Contraindicated in women with hypertension
  - Prostaglandin $F_2\alpha$ analogues (Hemabate) 0.25 mg IM repeated every 15 minutes as needed for up to eight doses. Contraindicated in those with asthma or bronchospasm
- **Manual tamponade of uterus**
  - Uterine packing—pack uterus with gauze with a sponge stick ending such that the gauze extends through the cervical os

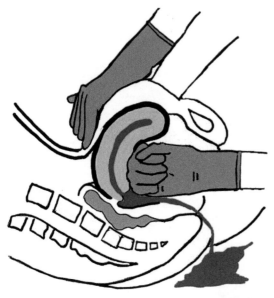

FIG. 17.3 Technique for bimanual massage. The provider places one hand in the patient's vagina and one hand externally. The uterus is compressed between the two hands.

- BAKRI[8] or other brand uterine balloons—insert balloon and instill 300–500 mL saline (Fig. 17.4)
- **Surgical approaches**
  - Uterine artery ligation[9]—a suture is placed around the uterine artery to decrease the pulse pressure within the uterus (Fig. 17.5)
  - B-lynch suture[10]—sutures are used to manually compress the uterus (Fig 17.6)
  - If these interventions fail, hysterectomy may be necessary

Fluid and Blood Product Replacement Therapy

- Ensure adequate IV access with two large bore IV lines, preferably 16 or 18 gauge
- Obtain baseline laboratory data including hemoglobin, hematocrit, platelets, and coagulation profile
- Begin infusion of colloid/crystalloid solution immediately (lactated Ringer's solution, normal saline, albumin, Hespan)

TABLE 17.1
Uterotonic Agents.

Medication	Dose	Route	Precautions
Oxytocin	40–80 units in 1 L normal saline	Intravenous	May cause free water retention. Avoid if there is hypotension
Misoprostol (Cytotec)	800–1000 mcg	Oral, sublingual, vaginal, or rectal	May cause fever, diarrhea
Methylergonovine (Methergine)	0.2 mg every 2–4 hours up to five doses	Intramuscular	Avoid in women with hypertension
Prostaglandin $F_2\alpha$ analogues (Hemabate)	0.25 mg every 15 minutes up to eight doses	Intramuscular	Avoid in women with asthma

(A)   **(B)**

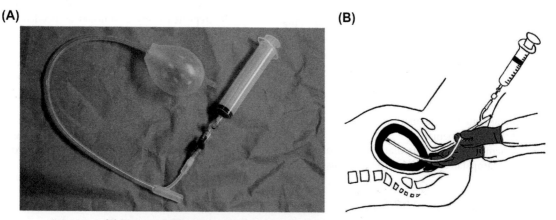

FIG. 17.4 **(A)** Photo and **(B)** placement of uterine balloon to provide manual tamponade of uterus.

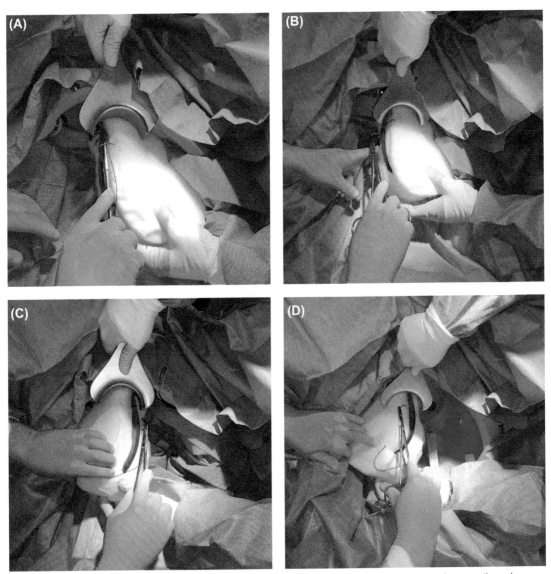

FIG. 17.5 Uterine artery ligation simulation. Suture is placed around the uterine vessels to decrease the pulse pressure of blood flow to the uterus. These figures show the O' Leary stitch training using foam material. The stitches are placed at the level of the internal os. **(A-B)** The operator is at the left of the manikin and the stitch is placed medially and anteriorly to the vessels and directed posteriorly and laterally to the vessels. **(C-D)** The stitch is placed posteriorly and laterally to the vessels and directed anteriorly and medially to the vessels.

- Monitor vital signs, urine output, and consider Foley catheter
- Keep the patient warm
- Order blood products in anticipation of transfusion. Verbal or written consent for transfusion should be obtained

- Transfusion of blood products should be initiated with signs of hemodynamic compromise such as hypotension and/or tachycardia
- If the situation is life threatening and does not allow for consent to be obtained, document appropriately in the medical record

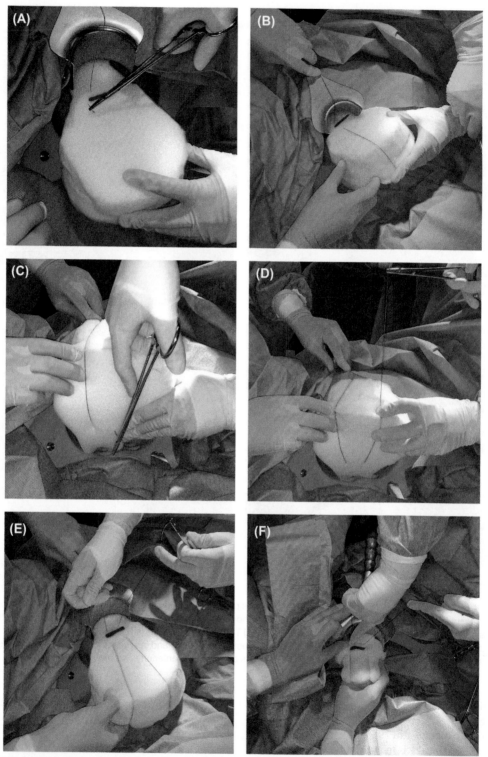

FIG. 17.6 B-lynch suture simulation. Beginning to the left side of the patient's uterus, **(A)** a stitch is placed anteriorly **(B)** and looped superiorly over the uterus. **(C)** The suture is then placed posteriorly from left to right. Finally, **(D)** the suture is brought superiorly over the uterus and **(E)** secured anteriorly on the right of the uterus. **(F)** When the suture is tied, it is used to compress the uterus.

REFERENCES

1. Committee on Practice B-O. Practice bulletin No. 183: postpartum hemorrhage. *Obstet Gynecol.* 2017;130(4):e168−e186.

2. Sebghati M, Chandraharan E. An update on the risk factors for and management of obstetric haemorrhage. *Womens Health (Lond).* 2017;13(2):34−40.

3. Butwick AJ, Ramachandran B, Hegde P, Riley ET, El-Sayed YY, Nelson LM. Risk Factors for Severe Postpartum Hemorrhage After Cesarean Delivery: Case-Control Studies. *Anesth Analg.* 2017;125(2):523−532.

4. Nyfløt LT, Sandven I, Stray-Pedersen B, Pettersen S, Al-Zirqi I, Rosenberg M, Jacobsen AF, Vangen S. Risk factors for severe postpartum hemorrhage: a case-control study. *BMC Pregnancy Childbirth.* 2017;17(1):17.

5. Dionne MD, Deneux-Tharaux C, Dupont C, Basso O, Rudigoz RC, Bouvier-Colle MH, Le Ray C. Duration of Expulsive Efforts and Risk of Postpartum Hemorrhage in Nulliparous Women: A Population-Based Study. *PLoS One.* 2015;10(11):e0142171.

6. Zuckerwise LC, Pettker CM, Illuzzi J, Raab CR, Lipkind HS. Use of a novel visual aid to improve estimation of obstetric blood loss. *Obstet Gynecol.* 2014;123(5):982−986.

7. Hofmeyr GJ, Abdel-Aleem H, Abdel-Aleem MA. Uterine massage for preventing postpartum haemorrhage. *Cochrane Database Syst Rev.* 2008;(3).

8. Bakri Y, Amri A, Abdul Jabbar F. Tamponade-balloon for obstetrical bleeding. *Int J Gynaecol Obstetrics.* 2001;74(2):139−142.

9. O'Leary JL, O'Leary JA. Uterine artery ligation in the control of intractable postpartum hemorrhage. *Am J Obstet Gynecol.* 1966;94(7):920−924.

10. B-Lynch C, Coker A, Lawal AH, Abu J, Cowen MJ. The B-Lynch surgical technique for the control of massive postpartum haemorrhage: an alternative to hysterectomy? Five cases reported. *Br J Obstet Gynaecol.* 1997;104(3):372−375.

Postpartum Hemorrhage Simulation

MATERIALS NEEDED
- Manikin or volunteer to act as standardized patient

KEY PERSONNEL
- Anesthesiologist
- Attending obstetrician
- Operating room staff
- Resident physician (if available in your institution)
- Two nurses

SAMPLE SCENARIO
A 36-year-old G7P6006 is resting comfortably after giving birth to a healthy 7lb 15oz (3600 g) infant. Her labor lasted 20 hours. The placenta was delivered intact. Forty-five minutes after the birth, the nurse assesses the uterine fundus and finds it boggy. There is blood pooling underneath the woman's perineum and buttocks.

DEBRIEFING AND DOCUMENTATION
- Etiology of hemorrhage
- Quantitative blood loss
- Steps taken to control hemorrhage
- IV fluids, blood products received
- Plan for monitoring
- Communication with patient and family

Simulation Checklist

		Time	Comments
Call for help	Emergency call bell		
	Clearly stated the problem		
	Requested specific personnel and supplies		
	Activated the hemorrhage protocol		
Airway	Maintained airway		
Breathing	Checked breathing		
	Administered high flow O_2 via nonrebreather		
	Positioned patient flat or head down		
Circulation	Inserted IV cannula (needs two large bore IVs)		
	Took blood pressure		
	Drew blood for CBC, PT, PTT, fibrinogen, BMP, and calcium		
	Requested blood—considered giving O negative if indicated		
Examination	Measured blood loss		
	Assessed uterine tone		
	Inspected placenta		
	Checked for lacerations		
Monitoring	Blood pressure		
	Respirations/oxygen saturation		
	Urine output		
Interventions	Oxytocin infusion		
	Misoprostol 800–1000 mcg		
	Hemabate 0.25 mg IM q15 minutes (Max 8 doses)		
	Methergine 0.2 mg IM q2 hours		
	Considered Bakri balloon		
Documentation	Timing of events		
	Medication administered		
	Persons present		
Communication	Call-out		
	Directed communication		
	Closed-loop communication		

Technical Skills	Non-Technical Skills
List causes of postpartum hemorrhage	Use direct communication
Perform bimanual massage	Use closed-loop communication
List doses of uterotonic agents	Assign team roles
Perform surgical interventions for postpartum hemorrhage	Debrief with team

Let's debrief. . .

Technical and nontechnical skills for postpartum hemorrhage.

CHAPTER 18

Blood Transfusion

LEARNING OBJECTIVES

- Identify the contents and indications for various blood component therapies.
- Recognize and manage transfusion reactions.

In the event of a hemorrhage, blood transfusion can be lifesaving. The obstetric team must be well-versed in when to transfuse which products as well as how to respond to transfusion reactions (Fig. 18.1).

BLOOD COMPONENTS[1]

Tables 18.1 shows the components of blood products and the expected clinical response to each product.

MASSIVE BLOOD TRANSFUSION[1-9]

- Historically defined by transfusion of 10 or more units of red blood cells (RBCs) in 24 hours
- Outcomes may be improved by early initiation of fresh frozen plasma (FFP) and platelets (but data limited in obstetric patients)
- Best practices recommend following institutional protocols for massive transfusion—a common ratio is 1:1:1 of packed red blood cells:fresh frozen plasma:platelets
  - Remember, a superpack of platelets is actually 4–6 units of platelets.
- The following labs should be monitored during massive transfusion:
  - INR—if >1.5, give 2 units FFP
  - Platelets—if <100 K, give one superpack platelets
  - Fibrinogen—if <100 mg/dL, give two pooled bags cryoprecipitate
  - Potassium (K+)—if >5 mEq/L, give 500 mL D10 + 10 units of regular insulin over 60 minutes AND give 1 g of calcium gluconate over slow IV infusion
  - Ionized calcium—if <1 mmol/L, give 1 g of calcium gluconate

TRANSFUSION REACTIONS[2,6]
Acute Hemolytic Reaction[10]

- Symptoms
  - Fever
  - Hypotension
  - Hematuria
  - Wheezing
- Treatment
  - Stop transfusion
  - Send blood and sample of patient's blood to blood bank
  - Bolus crystalloid fluids ($3L/m^2/24$ hours)
  - Consider dopamine 1–5 mcg/kg/min
  - Consider 20g of mannitol given as 20% solution
  - Repeat mannitol if urine output is <100 ml/hr for two or more hours

Tranfusion-Related Acute Lung Injury

- Symptoms
  - Shortness of breath
  - Hypoxemia
  - Rales
- Treatment
  - Stop transfusion
  - Apply oxygen
  - Consider need for mechanical ventilation

Allergy

- Symptoms
  - Shortness of breath
  - Wheezing
  - Hives
- Treatment
  - Diphenhydramine 25–100 mg IV or PO

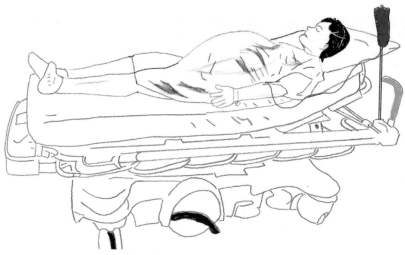

Acute Hemolytic Reaction	Bacterial contamination	Allergy	Transfusion Related Acute Lung Injury
Fever	High fever	Shortness of breath	Shortness of breath
Hypotension	Shock	Wheezing	Hypoxemia
Hematuria	Tachycardia	Hives	Rales
Wheezing			

FIG. 18.1 Symptoms of transfusion reaction.

TABLE 18.1
Blood Components

Blood Product	Contents	Volume	Expected Effect
Packed red blood cells (RBCs)[2]	Red blood cells	250–350 mL	Raise hemoglobin by 1 g/dL
Platelets (given as "superpack" of 6 units)[3]	Platelets	250–300 mL	Raise platelets by 30,000/mm³
Fresh frozen plasma (FFP)[4]	All clotting factors	200–300 mL	Raise fibrinogen by 8–10 mg/dL
Cryoprecipitate (given as pool of five bags)[4]	Fibrinogen, vWF, factor VIII, factor XIII	100 mL	Raise fibrinogen by 50 mg/dL

Bacterial Contamination[12]

- Symptoms
  - High fever
  - Shock
  - Tachycardia
- Treatment
  - Stop transfusion
  - Save transfusion materials for cultures
  - Initiate broad-spectrum antibiotics

Volume Overload[13]

- Symptoms
  - Shortness of breath, worse when lying down
  - Rales
  - Tachycardia
  - Distended jugular veins
- Treatment
  - Stop transfusion
  - Apply oxygen
  - Furosemide

REFERENCES

1. Klein AA, Arnold P, Bingham RM, et al. AAGBI guidelines: the use of blood components and their alternatives 2016. *Anaesthesia*. 2016;71(7):829–842.
2. Osterman JL, Arora S. Blood product transfusions and reactions. *Hematol Oncol Clin North Am*. 2017;31(6): 1159–1170.
3. Slichter SJ. Platelet transfusion therapy. *Hematol Oncol Clin North Am*. 2007;21(4):697–729.
4. De Backer D, Vandekerckhove B, Stanworth S, Williamson L, Hermans C, Van der Linden P, Hübner R, Baele P, Jochmans K, Ferrant A, Lambermont M, Muylle L, Toungouz M. Guidelines for the use of fresh frozen plasma. *Acta Clin Belg*. 2008;63(6):381–390.
5. Nascimento B, Goodnough LT, Levy JH. Cryoprecipitate therapy. *Br J Anaesth*. 2014;113(6):922–934.
6. Delaney M, Wendel S, Bercovitz RS, et al. Transfusion reactions: prevention, diagnosis, and treatment. *Lancet (London, England)*. 2016;388(10061):2825–2836.
7. Pacheco LD, Saade GR, Costantine MM, Clark SL, Hankins GD. An update on the use of massive transfusion protocols in obstetrics. *Am J Obstet Gynecol*. 2016;214(3): 340–344.
8. Hodgman EI, Cripps MW, Mina MJ, Bulger EM, Schreiber MA, Brasel KJ, Cohen MJ, Muskat P, Myers JG, Alarcon LH, Rahbar MH, Holcomb JB, Cotton BA, Fox EE, Del Junco DJ, Wade CE, Phelan HA, PROMMTT Study Group. External validation of a smartphone app model to predict the need for massive transfusion using five different definitions. *J Trauma Acute Care Surg*. 2018; 84(2):397–402.
9. McQuilten ZK, Crighton G, Brunskill S, Morison JK, Richter TH, Waters N, Murphy MF, Wood EM. Optimal dose, timing and ratio of blood products in massive transfusion: results from a systematic review. *Transfus Med Rev*. 2018;32(1):6.
10. Greenwalt TJ. Pathogenesis and management of hemolytic transfusion reactions. *Semin Hematol*. 1981;18(2):84–94.
11. Bux J, Sachs UJ. The pathogenesis of transfusion-related acute lung injury (TRALI). *Br J Haematol*. 2007;136: 788–799.
12. Palavecino EL, Yomtovian RA, Jacobs MR. Bacterial contamination of platelets. *Transfus Apher Sci*. 2010;42:71–82.
13. Gajic O, Gropper MA, Hubmayr RD. Pulmonary edema after transfusion: how to differentiate transfusion-associated circulatory overload from transfusion-related acute lung injury. *Crit Care Med*. 2006;34:S109–S113.

Blood Transfusion Simulation

MATERIALS NEEDED
- Manikin or volunteer to act as standardized patient

KEY PERSONNEL
- Attending obstetrician
- Nurse
- Resident physician (if available in your institution)

SAMPLE SCENARIO
A 23-year-old woman is postpartum day 1 from a vaginal delivery complicated by postpartum hemorrhage. She complains of dizziness and headache. Her hemoglobin is 5.4 g/dL. After discussing the risks and benefits with the patient, you decide to proceed with transfusion of 2 units of packed red blood cells. Review your institutional procedures and safety mechanisms for blood transfusion.

The nurse hangs the first unit of packed red blood cells. After 15 minutes, the patient's temperature rises to 38.6 C. The patient complains of shortness of breath. How do you proceed?

DEBRIEFING AND DOCUMENTATION
- Time transfusion reaction noted
- Time transfusion stopped
- Was blood bank notified
- Interventions
- Current patient condition

Simulation Checklist

		Time	Comments
Initial response	Recognized transfusion reaction		
	Stopped blood transfusion		
	Notified physician		
Airway	Checked for airway compromise, anaphylaxis		
Breathing	Checked breathing		
Circulation	Maintained patency of IV with normal saline		
	Took blood pressure		
Interventions	Checked urine for hematuria		
	Sent sample of patient's blood to blood bank		
	Bolused normal saline		
Documentation	Timing of events		
	Notification of blood bank		
	Persons present		
Communication	Directed communication		
	Closed-loop communication		

Technical Skills	Non-Technical Skills
Describe available blood products and their indications	Communicate with blood bank and other team members
Obtain IV access with proper blood tubing	Communicate with patient
Perform blood transfusion safety checks	Refer to institutional guidelines for transfusion policy
List potential blood transfusion reactions	Debrief with team

Let's debrief. . .

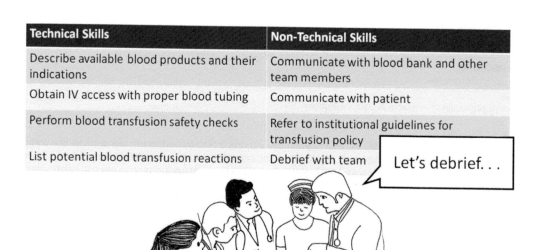

Technical and nontechnical skills for blood transfusion.

Uterine Inversion

Uterine inversion occurs when the fundus of the uterus collapses after delivery and, in its most severe form, delivers through the vagina (Fig. 19.1 A-B)[1,2]. If not quickly recognized, it has a reported maternal mortality rate as high as 15%.[3]

RISK FACTORS[3,4]

- Fundal placenta
- Uterine atony (or use of medications such as magnesium that reduce uterine tone)
- Placenta accreta
- Short cord
- Connective tissue disorders

DIAGNOSIS[3,5]

Complete uterine inversion is easily diagnosed by palpation of the uterine fundus within or beyond the vaginal introitus. More subtle cases of uterine inversion can be diagnosed by heavy postpartum bleeding with a nonpalpable uterine fundus. Uterine inversion can also be visualized sonographically with the inverted fundus directed caudally instead of the usual cephalad orientation.

MANAGEMENT[3]

The priority in management is to replace the uterine fundus to its correct anatomic position (Table 19.1).

Initial Steps

- Call for help!! Necessary personnel include the following:
  - An experienced care provider
  - Two labor and delivery nurses
  - An anesthesiologist
  - Operating room staff
- State clearly "There is a uterine inversion."
- Insure IV access with large bore IV
- Stop all uterotonic medications
- Consider uterine relaxant
  - Terbutaline 0.25 mg subcutaneously
  - *OR* nitroglycerin 50–500 mcg intravenously in aliquots of 50–100 mcg
  - Halothane general anesthesia
- Perform maneuvers as described below to restore uterus to anatomic location
- Do not remove placenta until after uterus is replaced—this may increase blood loss
- Resuscitate with fluids, blood products as needed
- Once uterus replaced, administer uterotonics

Johnson Maneuver (Fig. 19.2)[7]

- Place fingers on uterine fundus
- Apply pressure to the inverted fundus, thus pushing it through the cervical ring
- Use the "last out, first in" approach—replace what is normally the most distal part of the uterus first and work your way to the fundus

Hydrostatic Pressure (Fig. 19.3)[8]

- Hang a bag of warmed fluid on an IV pole above the level of the patient
- Hold the IV tubing in the vagina
- Allow the fluid to fill the vagina and allow the pressure to correct the uterine inversion

Huntington Procedure (Fig. 19.4)[9]

- If unable to replace the uterus vaginally, perform laparotomy

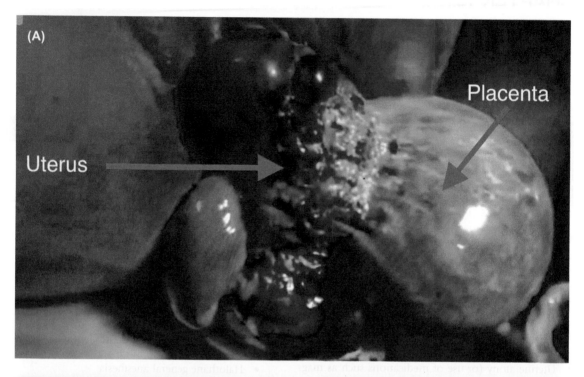

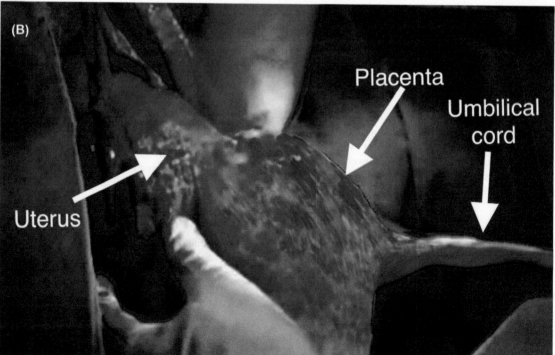

FIG. 19.1 Uterine inversion with placenta **(A)**; Uterine inversion with placenta and umbilical cord **(B)**.

- Locate the cup of the uterus formed by the inversion
- Grasp the round ligaments with Allis clamps and apply gentle upward traction
- As more of the round ligament becomes visible, reposition clamps closer to the fundus of the uterus
- Continue clamping and providing traction until inversion is corrected.

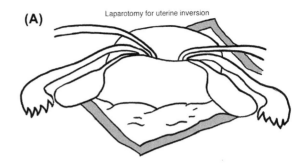

(A)   Laparotomy for uterine inversion

TABLE 19.1

Stepwise Maneuvers for Uterine Inversion

- Manual replacement of uterus with fist/fingers
- Transvaginal hydrostatic pressure
- Perform laparotomy
- Replacement of uterus with traction on round ligaments
- Posterior colpotomy with digital replacement of uterus

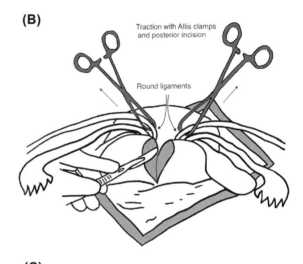

(B)   Traction with Allis clamps and posterior incision

Round ligaments

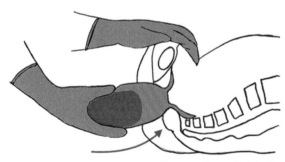

FIG. 19.2 Johnson maneuver. Pressure is applied to the inverted uterus to replace it to its anatomic position.

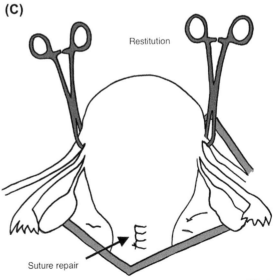

(C)   Restitution

Suture repair

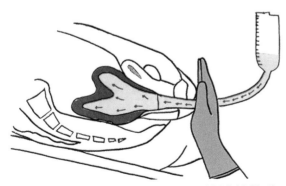

FIG. 19.3 Hydrostatic pressure. Warmed IV fluid fills the vagina and provides hydrostatic pressure to replace the uterus.

FIG. 19.4 Huntington and Haultaim procedures. **(A)** A laparotomy is made and **(B)** allis clamps are used to place traction on the round ligaments. If necessary, a posterior hysterotomy is used to facilitate repositioning the uterus. **(C)** Shows the repositioned uterus.

Haultain Procedure[10]

- This procedure also requires a laparotomy
- Locate the cup of the uterus formed by the inversion

- Incise the posterior portion of the inversion ring (Fig. 19.4)
- Insert fingers through incision and reposition the uterus to its correct anatomic position
- Repair the hysterotomy incision

(A)

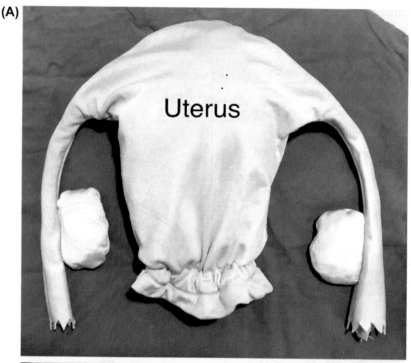

(B)

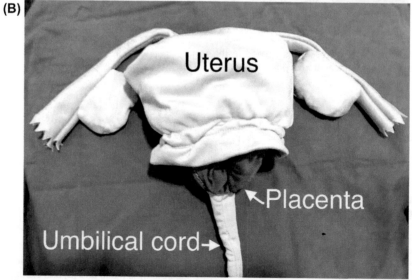

FIG. 19.5 Model used at for the simulation of uterine inversion. A: Normal uterus with tubes and ovaries (white); B: Uterine inversion. This model is placed inside the pelvis and the uterine inversion is simulated. This model was created by Dr.Genxia Li at Zhengzhou University

REFERENCES

1. Bhalla R, Wuntakal R, Odejinmi F, Khan RU. Acute inversion of the uterus. *Obstet Gynaecol.* 2009;11(1):13−18.
2. O'Sullivan JV. Acute inversion of the uterus. *Br Med J.* 1945;2(4417):282.
3. Hostetler DR, Bosworth MF. Uterine inversion: a life-threatening obstetric emergency. *J Am Board Fam Pract.* 2000;13(2):120−123.
4. Baskett TF. Acute uterine inversion: a review of 40 cases. *J Obstet Gynaecol Can.* 2002;24(12):953−956.
5. Smulian JC, DeFulvio JD, Diven L, Terrazas JL. Sonographic findings in acute uterine inversion. *J Clin Ultrasound.* 2013;41(7):453−456.
6. Dayan SS, Schwalbe SS. The use of small-dose intravenous nitroglycerin in a case of uterine inversion. *Anesth Analg.* 1996 May;82(5):1091−1093.
7. Johnson AB. A new concept in the replacement of the inverted uterus and a report of nine cases. *Am J Obstet Gynecol.* 1949;57(3):557−562.
8. Momani AW, Hassan A. Treatment of puerperal uterine inversion by the hydrostatic method; reports of five cases. *Eur J Obstet Gynecol Reprod Biol.* 1989;32(3):281−285.
9. Huntington JL, Irving FC, Kellogg FS. Abdominal reposition in acute inversion of the puerperal uterus. *Am J Obstet Gynecol.* 1928;15(1):34−40.
10. Haultain FJ. The treatment of chronic uterine inversion by abdominal hysterotomy, with a successful case. *Br Med J.* 1901:974−976.

Uterine Inversion Simulation

MATERIALS NEEDED
- Pelvic model with uterus (Fig. 19.5 A-B)

KEY PERSONNEL
- Anesthesiologist
- Attending obstetrician
- Nurse
- Operating room staff
- Resident physician (if available in your institution)

SAMPLE SCENARIO
Maria is a 38-year-old G6P6 who just delivered at healthy 7# infant. Despite application of traction on the umbilical cord, there is difficulty delivering the placenta. You note significant vaginal bleeding and a firm bulge in the patient's vagina.

DEBRIEFING AND DOCUMENTATION
- Time diagnosis made
- Uterine relaxants given
- Maneuvers used
- Time uterus replaced
- Blood loss
- Fluids received
- Uterotonics given after uterine replacement

Simulation Checklist

		Time	Comments
Call for help	Emergency call bell		
	Clearly stated the problem		
	Requested specific personnel and supplies		
Circulation	Inserted IV cannula (needs 2 large bore IV's)		
	Took blood pressure		
	Requested blood—considered giving O negative if indicated		
	Measured blood loss		
Replacement of uterus	Stopped uterotonics		
	Considered uterine relaxant: • Terbutaline 0.25 mg SQ • Nitroglycerin 50–500 mcg IV in aliquots of 50–100 mcg • Halothane general anesthesia		
	Placenta left in situ until uterus replaced		
	Attempted to manually replace uterus		
	If necessary, consideration given to laparotomy		
	Uterotonics given after uterus replaced		
Documentation	Timing of events		
	Medication administered		
	Persons present		
Communication	Call-out		
	Directed communication		
	Closed-loop communication		

Technical Skills	Non-Technical Skills
List risk factors for uterine inversion	Assign team roles
Perform vaginal replacement of inverted uterus	Use closed loop communication
Perform laparotomy for replacement of inverted uterus	Communicate with patient

Let's debrief. . .

Technical and nontechnical skills for uterine inversion.

CHAPTER 20

Hypertensive Urgency and Eclampsia

LEARNING OBJECTIVES

- Recognize the presentation of eclampsia.
- Describe management priorities for a patient with eclampsia.

Eclampsia is defined as new-onset, generalized, tonic-clonic seizures or coma in a patient with preeclampsia. It is one of the several clinical manifestations of severe preeclampsia. Preeclampsia/eclampsia constitutes a common cause of maternal morbidity and mortality (Fig. 20.1)[1,2].

RISK FACTORS[2,3]

- Primiparity
- Personal or family history of preeclampsia or eclampsia
- Chronic hypertension
- Chronic renal disease
- History of thrombophilia
- Multifetal gestation
- In vitro fertilization
- Diabetes mellitus
- Obesity
- System lupus erythematosus
- Advanced maternal age

Seizure Stroke Posterior reversible encephalopathy	Pulmonary edema	Renal failure Proteinuria	Hemolysis Thrombocytopenia Disseminated intravascular coagulation
	Liver failure Subcapsular hematoma	Placental abruption	

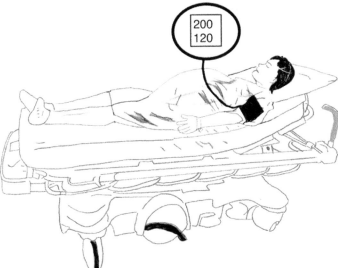

FIG. 20.1 Organ systems affected by preeclampsia.

DIAGNOSIS[4]

Eclampsia is defined by new-onset grand mal seizures in a patient with preeclampsia. Diagnostic criteria for preeclampsia are as follows:

- Hypertension (BP greater than or equal to 140/90 on two occasions at least 4 hours apart) *AND*
- Proteinuria (more than 300 mg protein in 24-hour collection *or* protein:creatinine ratio greater than or equal to 0.3)
- In the absence of proteinuria, preeclampsia can still be diagnosed if there is new-onset hypertension and any one or more of the following:
  - Platelet count less than 100 K/μL
  - Serum creatinine greater than 1.1 mg/dL or twice baseline (in the absence of other renal disease)
  - Liver transaminases elevated to twice normal
  - Pulmonary edema
  - Cerebral or visual symptoms

MANAGEMENT
Supportive Care

- Most eclamptic seizures are self-limited
- Priority is protecting the mother's airway, securing airway patency, and preventing recurrent seizures (Fig. 20.2)
- The patient should be placed in a left lateral position

- Supplemental oxygen (8–10 L/minutes) via non-rebreather face mask
- Suction should be available if needed to prevent aspiration
- Arrange environment to reduce risk from seizure (i.e., raise and pad bed rails, etc.)

Treatment of Hypertension[5]

Antihypertensive therapy should be initiated for sustained systolic blood pressures $\geq$160 mmHg or diastolic pressures greater than 105–110 mmHg. Options for IV control of blood pressure include the following:

- Labetalol—begin with 20 mg IV push over 2 minutes. If no response after 10 minutes, escalate doses sequentially to 40, 80 mg (Fig. 20.3)
- Hydralazine—begin with 5–10 mg IV push over 2 minutes. If no response after 20 minutes, administer additional 10 mg IV (Fig. 20.4)
- If IV access is not available, patient may be treated with the following:
- Nifedipine—begin with 10 mg PO. If no response in 20 minutes, give 20 mg PO. If no response in 20 minutes, repeat 20 mg PO. If no response in 20 minutes, switch to labetalol 20 mg IV (Fig. 20.5)
- Rarely, blood pressure remains elevated despite the above treatment. In this case, an IV drip such as

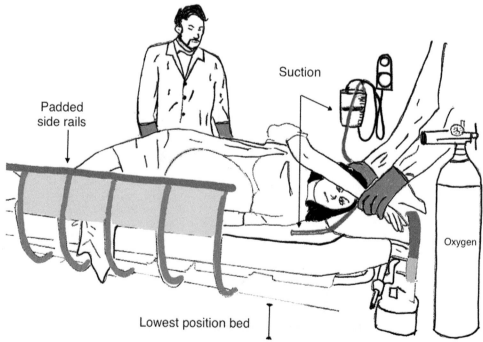

FIG. 20.2 Supportive care during eclamptic seizure. Priority should be given to protecting patient and her airway during seizure and initiating magnesium sulfate to prevent recurrent seizures.

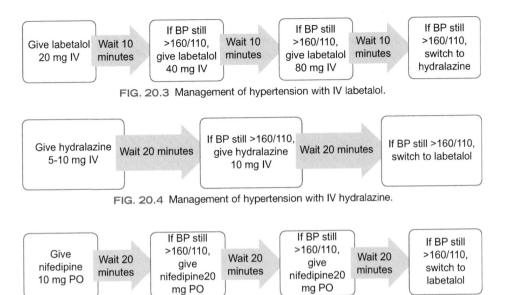

FIG. 20.3 Management of hypertension with IV labetalol.

FIG. 20.4 Management of hypertension with IV hydralazine.

FIG. 20.5 Management of hypertension with PO nifedipine.

nicardipine is initiated with the help of the anesthesiologist

Prevention of Recurrent Seizures

Preferred medication for seizure prevention is magnesium sulfate as outlined in Table 20.1[6]

- **Loading dose** is 4—6 g IV over 15—20 minutes
- **Maintenance dose is** 2 g/hour as a continuous IV infusion
- If patient does not have IV access, give an initial dose of 5 g IM into each buttock (10 g total) followed by 5 g intramuscularly every 4 hours
- Patients on magnesium sulfate should be monitored closely for signs of toxicity (Table 20.2)
  - Respirations >12 per minute, normal patellar reflexes, and urine output >100 mL in 4 hours indicate absence of toxicity—following the serum magnesium level is not necessary
- In case of toxicity, stop the magnesium. Calcium gluconate (1 g IV) is the antidote for magnesium toxicity
- Extra precautions with magnesium sulfate should be taken as follows:
  - In patients with renal insufficiency, maintenance dosing should be lower; serum magnesium concentration should be 4.8—8.4 mg/dL (1.9—3.5 mmol/L)
  - Concomitant use of magnesium sulfate and calcium channel blockers may result in hypotension, but the risk seems to be minimal
  - Magnesium sulfate is contraindicated in women with myasthenia gravis

TABLE 20.1
Medications for Magnesium-Resistant Seizures

Medication	Dose	Precautions
Magnesium sulfate	6 g load followed by 2 g/hour maintenance; give additional 2 g over 5—10 minutes for recurrent seizures	Contraindicated with myasthenia gravis and hypocalcemia; use with caution in renal failure; monitor for signs of toxicity
Diazepam	5—10 mg IV	Maximum dose 30 mg
Lorazepam	4 mg IV over at least 2 minutes	—
Midazolam	1—2 mg every 5 minutes	Maximum dose 2 mg/kg

TABLE 20.2
Signs of Magnesium Toxicity

Loss of deep tendon reflexes
Decreased level of consciousness
Respiratory depression
Cardiac arrest

Recurrent Seizures

- An additional bolus of 2 g magnesium sulfate over 5–10 minutes is attempted first, with frequent monitoring for signs of magnesium toxicity
- If two such boluses do not control seizures, then other drugs should be given
  - Diazepam: 5–10 mg IV every 5–10 minutes at a rate ≤5 mg/minutes and maximum dose 30 mg
  - Lorazepam: 4 mg IV at maximum rate 2 mg/minutes
  - Midazolam: 1–2 mg bolus IV at a rate of 2 mg/minutes. Additional boluses can be given every 5 minutes until seizures stop (up to a maximum of 2 mg/kg)

Fetal Monitoring

- Priority should be stabilizing mother
- Fetal bradycardia lasting at least 3–5 minutes is a common finding during and immediately after an eclamptic seizure
- If the fetal heart rate tracing does not improve within 10–15 minutes of maternal stabilization, consider the possibility of an abruption and perform a cesarean

Evaluation for Prompt Delivery

- Treatment for eclampsia is prompt delivery *after maternal stabilization*

- Does not necessarily require cesarean delivery. Factors to consider:
  - Gestational age
  - Cervical status
  - If patient is in labor
  - Fetal position
  - Fetal condition
- Induction is a reasonable option for pregnancies at least 32–34 weeks of gestation and for earlier gestations with a favorable Bishop score

REFERENCES

1. Bokslag A, van Weissenbruch M, Mol BW, de Groot CJ. Preeclampsia; short and long-term consequences for mother and neonate. *Early Hum Dev.* 2016;102:47–50.
2. Ghulmiyyah L, Sibai B. Maternal mortality from preeclampsia/eclampsia. *Semin Perinatol.* 2012;36(1):56–59.
3. Committee opinion No. 638: first-trimester risk assessment for early-onset preeclampsia. *Obstet Gynecol.* 2015;126(3):e25–e27.
4. American College of Obstetricians and Gynecologists. *Hypertension in Pregnancy.* 2013 (Washington DC).
5. Committee on Obstetric Practice. Committee opinion No. 692: emergent therapy for acute-onset, severe hypertension during pregnancy and the postpartum period. *Obstet Gynecol.* 2017;129(4):e90–e95.
6. Sibai BM. Diagnosis, prevention, and management of eclampsia. *Obstet Gynecol.* 2005;105(2):402–410.

Hypertensive Urgency Simulation

MATERIALS NEEDED
- Manikin or volunteer to act as standardized patient

KEY PERSONNEL
- Attending obstetrician
- Resident physician (if available in your institution)
- Two nurses

SAMPLE SCENARIO
A 20-year-old G1 P0 presents at 38 weeks 0 days complaining of a moderate bilateral occipital headache and decreased fetal movement. Her prenatal course was unremarkable until last week when her blood pressure increased from a baseline of 110/60 to 135/85. Her urine dip stick was 1 + during that visit. She was asked to complete a 24-hour urine collection for total protein at home and get a biophysical profile. She has done neither. On presentation, her BP is 185/105, P 95, RR 20, and T99.4. FHT is reassuring.

DEBRIEFING AND DOCUMENTATION
- Initial vital signs
- Urine dipstick
- Laboratory results
- Medications given
- Current maternal, fetal status
- Seizure precautions initiated
- Plan for monitoring/management
- Communication with patient and family

Simulation Checklist		Time	Comments
Initial nursing assessment	Checked vital signs		
	Continuous fetal monitoring		
	Called for help		
	Started IV		
	Drew blood work		
Initial provider assessment	Confirmed blood pressure		
	Focused history		
	Focused exam		
	Ordered CBC, CMP, spot urine protein:creatinine ratio, possible LDH, uric acid, PT, PTT, fibrinogen, and/or urine tox		
	Communicated up the chain of command		
Medications	Antihypertensive medications: Labetalol 20/40/80/80 mg or hydralazine 5—10/10 mg		
	Magnesium sulfate 6 g load followed by 2 g/hour		
	Betamethasone (if preterm)		
Other interventions	Total IV fluids 100—125 mL/hour		
	Placed Foley catheter		
	Raised and padded side rails		
	DVT prophylaxis		
	Discussed urgency of delivery		
Documentation	Vital signs		
	Timing of medications		
Communication	SBAR technique		
	Directed communication		
	Closed-loop communication		

Technical Skills	Non-Technical Skills
List diagnostic criteria for preeclampsia	Use direct communication
List medications and doses for hypertension in pregnancy	Provide low-stimulation environment for patients with preeclampsia
List medications and doses for seizure prophylaxis	Prioritize maternal resuscitation during seizure
Provide supportive care during seizure	Debrief with team

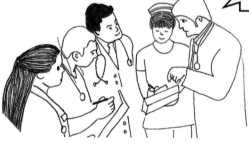

Technical and non-technical skills for eclampsia.

Sepsis

DEFINITIONS

Systemic Inflammatory Response Syndromes (SIRS)

Defined by two or more of the following:

- Temperature >38 or <36°C
- Heart rate >90 beats per minute
- Respiratory rate >20 breaths/minute or $PaCO_2$ <32 mmHg
- White blood cells >12,000 cells/mm^3 or <4000 cells/mm^3 or >10% bands[1,2]

Sepsis

Defined by SIRS with a source of infection.

Severe Sepsis

Defined by sepsis with end organ dysfunction (Fig. 21.1).

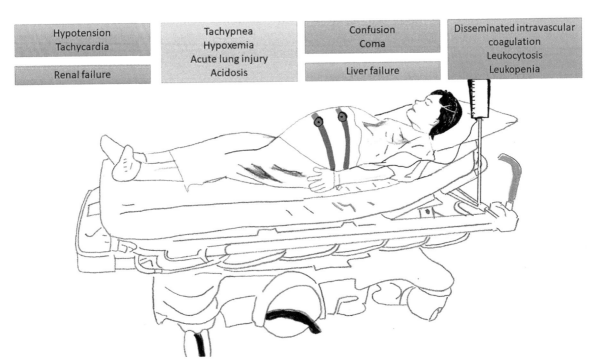

FIG. 21.1 Maternal sepsis can result in multisystem organ failure.

Safety Training for Obstetric Emergencies. https://doi.org/10.1016/B978-0-323-69672-2.00021-7

SURVIVING SEPSIS GUIDELINES

- Within first 3 hours
  - Measure lactate level
  - Obtain blood cultures
  - Begin antibiotics
  - Resuscitate with 30 mL/kg crystalloid if mean arterial pressure $\leq$65 mmHg or lactate $\geq$ 4 mmol/L
- Within first 6 hours
  - Begin vasopressors if mean arterial pressure (MAP) does not respond to fluid boluses
    - Begin with norepinephrine 0.05–0.1 mcg/kg/minute and titrate up to 1 mcg/kg/minute for MAP $\geq$ 65 mmHg
  - If MAP does not respond to fluid boluses or initial lactate $\geq$ 4 mmol/L, measure central venous pressure and central venous oxygen saturation
  - Repeat lactate if initial measurement elevated[3,4]

CHOOSING ANTIMICROBIALS[3,5]

- Resistant Gram positives → Vancomycin, daptomycin, linezolid
- Resistant Gram negatives → Piperacillin/tazobactam, carbapenemases
- Cytomegalovirus → Valgancyclovir
- Fungal infections → Echinocandins, amphotericin B

REFERENCES

1. Chebbo A, et al. Maternal sepsis and septic shock. *Crit Care Clin.* 2016;32(1):119–135.
2. Parfitt SE, et al. Sepsis in obstetrics: pathophysiology and diagnostic definitions. *MCN Am J Matern Child Nurs.* 2017;42(4):194–198.
3. Barrier KM. Summary of the 2016 international surviving sepsis campaign: a clinician's guide. *Crit Care Nurs Clin N Am.* 2018;30(3):311–321.
4. Parfitt SE, Bogat ML, Roth C. Sepsis in obstetrics: treatment, prognosis, and prevention. *MCN Am J Matern Child Nurs.* 2017;42(4):206–209.
5. Plante LA. Management of sepsis and septic shock for the obstetrician-gynecologist. *Obstet Gynecol Clin N Am.* 2016; 43(4):659–678.

Sepsis Simulation

MATERIALS NEEDED
- Manikin or volunteer to act as standardized patient

KEY PERSONNEL
- Attending obstetrician
- Resident physician (if available in your institution)
- Two nurses

SAMPLE SCENARIO
A 25-year-old G3P2112 at 37 weeks 2 days gestation presents with abdominal pain, diarrhea, and decreased fetal movement. She was treated for a urinary tract infection 3 weeks ago. She states she has been leaking fluid for approximately 2 weeks. Speculum exam does not demonstrate any fluid. Her vitals are as follows: BP 90/60, HR 140, T 39.1, SpO$_2$ 99%.

DEBRIEFING AND DOCUMENTATION
- Potential sources of infection
- Systemic Inflammatory Response Syndrome criteria
- Evidence of organ dysfunction
- Initial resuscitation
- Antimicrobials
- Plan for ongoing monitoring and management
- Communication with patient and family

Simulation Checklist		Time	Comments
Initial response	Obtained history and physical		
	Obtained vital signs		
	Clearly stated the problem		
	Called for help		
	Requested specific personnel and supplies		
Airway	Checked for airway compromise		
Breathing	Checked breathing		
	Administered high-flow oxygen		
Circulation	Started 2 large-bore IVs		
	Collected blood for labs (including CBC, lactate, blood cultures)		
Interventions	IV fluids (30 mL/kg)		
	Oxygen		
	Broad spectrum antibiotics		
Monitoring	Blood pressure		
	Respirations		
	Oxygen saturation		
	Urinary output		
	Fetal heart rate (after mother stabilized)		
Documentation	Timing of events		
	Medications administered		
	Persons present		
Communication	Directed communication		
	Closed-loop communication		

Technical Skills	Non-Technical Skills
List criteria of systemic inflammatory response syndrome	Use direct communication
Describe guidelines for management of expected sepsis	Involve interdisciplinary team
Describe choice of antibiotic based on suspected infection	Communicate with patient

Technical and nontechnical skill sets with regards to maternal sepsis.

Diabetic Ketoacidosis

Diabetic ketoacidosis (DKA) is a relatively rare but life-threatening condition. Pregnant women are prone to develop more severe and more rapidly progressive episodes of DKA at lower glucose levels than nonpregnant women. In pregnancy, there is a particularly increased susceptibility to starvation, infection, and ketogenic factors.

RISK FACTORS[1]

- Vomiting
- Starvation
- Infections (urinary tract, respiratory tract, chorioamniotic infections, skin infections, dental infections, ENT infections, etc.)
- Poorly controlled glycemia (including noncompliance, insulin pump failure)
- Beta agonist use
- Steroid use
- Diabetic gastroparesis

DIAGNOSIS

- The signs and symptoms of diabetic ketoacidosis during pregnancy tend to develop faster than in the nonpregnant state. Signs and symptoms include the following (Fig. 22.1)[2,3]:
  - Hyperventilation/tachypnea or "Kussmaul respirations"
  - Tachycardia
  - Hypotension
  - Dehydration
  - Mental status changes with disorientation or coma

- Abnormal fetal heart tracing
- Polyuria or polydipsia
- Nausea or vomiting
- Abdominal pain or contractions
- Laboratory abnormalities (See Table 22.1)

TABLE 22.1
Laboratory Findings in DKA

Plasma glucose (usually)>250mg/dL
Anion gap>12mEq/L
Bicarbonate<15mEq/L
Arterial pH<7.30
Positive serum and urine ketones

MANAGEMENT

As detailed in Fig. 22.2, the management of DKA is aimed toward:
- Volume replacement/hydration
- Correction of hyperglycemia with insulin therapy
- Correction of electrolyte abnormalities and acidosis
- Correction of the underlying pathology/trigger

IV Fluid Replacement

- Start early IV access with two large bore catheters or central venous catheter
- Start fluid correction with normal saline
- Fluid deficit is corrected over 48 hours (75% in the initial 24 hours)

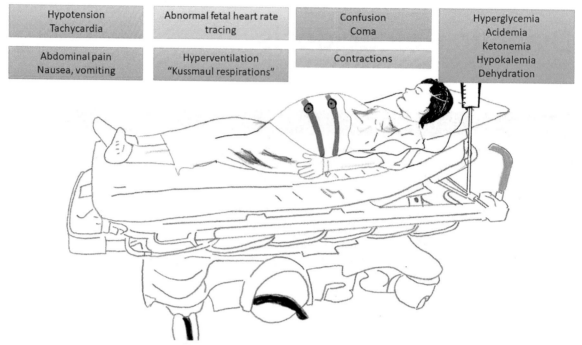

| Hypotension Tachycardia | Abnormal fetal heart rate tracing | Confusion Coma | Hyperglycemia Acidemia Ketonemia Hypokalemia Dehydration |
| Abdominal pain Nausea, vomiting | Hyperventilation "Kussmaul respirations" | Contractions | |

FIG. 22.1 Signs and symptoms of diabetic ketoacidosis.

- The total deficit is usually 100 mL/kg (6–10 L typically)
- Start isotonic normal saline at 1–2 L/h for 1–2 hours
- Continue isotonic normal saline at 250–500 ml/hr until glucose levels are under 250 mg/dL
- Once this glucose level is reached, continue an IV solution with 5% dextrose
- If hypernatremia is noted, switch solution to 0.45% saline and continue until hypernatremia is resolved
- Monitor closely during the initial 4 hours (hourly urine output, vital gas (VS) every 15 minutes)
- Monitor oxygen saturation continuously, providing supplemental O_2 as needed
- Monitor response with arterial blood gas (ABG), anion gap every 1–3 hours
- Investigate and treat precipitating factors simultaneously

Insulin Therapy

- *Do not give insulin until potassium known*
- Start IV with short-acting insulin: 8–10 unit bolus followed by 0.1 units/kg/hour

- Continue insulin until low serum bicarbonate, abnormal anion gap, and serum ketones are resolved (even if normal glycemia)
- Discontinue insulin IV infusion only after the first dose of SQ insulin is administered

Correction of Acidosis and Electrolyte Disturbances

- Correction of electrolyte imbalances, particularly hypokalemia, should start as soon as adequate renal function is documented
- The total potassium deficit is usually 5–10 mEq/L
- Correction of DKA typically causes intracellular shift of potassium
- Potassium level should be kept between 4 and 5 mEq/L. Potassium replacement is best accomplished with potassium chloride
- Phosphate replacement is only necessary when levels fall below 1 mg/dL, cardiac dysfunction ensues, or signs of obtundation are noted
- Phosphate is replaced with 10–20 mEq of potassium phosphate for each 10–20 mEq of potassium chloride

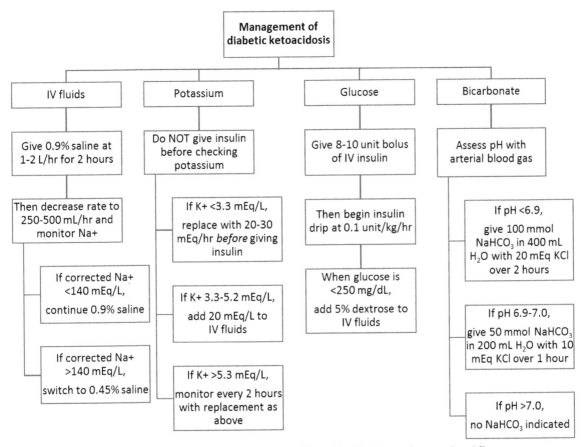

FIG. 22.2 Management of diabetic ketoacidosis (Modified from references 2 and 3).

- The need to replace other electrolytes is questionable. Some authors advocate replacement with pH below 7, cardiac dysfunction, sepsis, or shock
- Ketones should be followed serially

Fetal Monitoring

- Fetal heart rate monitoring during the acute episode of diabetic ketoacidosis often reveals minimal or absent variability, absent accelerations, and repetitive variable and late decelerations (Fig. 22.3). The fetal biophysical profile can also be abnormal,

and Doppler studies may show signs of blood flow redistribution (i.e., increased umbilical artery pulsatility index and reduced middle cerebral artery pulsatility index)
- It may take 4–8 hours for the fetal heart rate tracing to become normal
- Mortality and morbidity may be increased by cesarean delivery. DKA alone is not an indication for delivery. It is critical to stabilize the maternal condition before consideration, as this will often improve fetal status. If the condition does not improve despite aggressive DKA management, delivery may be indicated

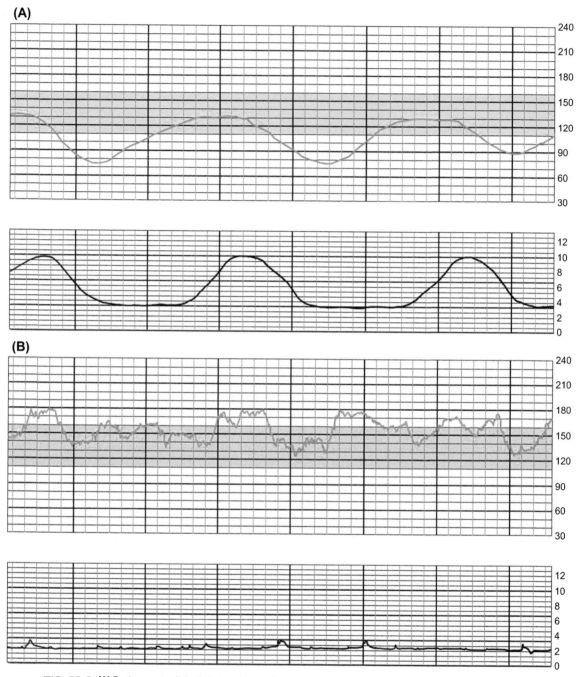

FIG. 22.3 **(A)** During acute diabetic ketoacidosis, fetal decelerations are common. **(B)** After resuscitation, the fetal heart rate tracing usually becomes reassuring.

REFERENCES

1. Dalfra MG, et al. Ketoacidosis in diabetic pregnancy. *J Matern Fetal Neonatal Med.* 2016;29(17):2889–2895.
2. de Veciana M. Diabetes ketoacidosis in pregnancy. *Semin Perinatol.* 2013;37(4):267–273.
3. Pregestational diabetes mellitus. ACOG Practice Bulletin No. 201. American College of Obstetricians and Gynecologists. *Obstet Gynecol.* 2018;132:e228–248.
4. Bryant SN, et al. Diabetic ketoacidosis complicating pregnancy. *J Neonatal Perinat Med.* 2017;10(1):17–23.

Diabetic Ketoacidosis Simulation

MATERIALS NEEDED
- Volunteer to act as standardized patient

KEY PERSONNEL
- Attending obstetrician
- Nurse
- Resident physician (if available in your institution)

SAMPLE SCENARIO
A 22-year-old G1P0 at 26 weeks gestation presents to labor and delivery. The patient has a known history of Type I diabetes mellitus since age 11. She states she has not taken her insulin for the last 2 days because she has had nausea and vomiting and has not been eating much. She now complains of worsening vomiting and abdominal pain. Her fingerstick BGT is 324.
What other history and physical would you perform?
What is your first priority in treating this patient?
What lab work would you like to test?

Bloodwork is remarkable for the following:
- Serum glucose 336 mg/dL
- Sodium 136 mEq/L
- Potassium 3.6 mEq/L
- Bicarbonate 12 mEq/L
- Anion gap 16 mEq/L
- pH 7.22

Explain your strategies for the following:
- IV fluid replacement
- Potassium replacement
- Blood glucose control
- pH management
- Fetal monitoring
- Repeating bloodwork

DEBRIEFING AND DOCUMENTATION
- Suspected precipitating factor for DKA
- Total fluid, electrolyte, insulin replacement received
- Plan for transitioning to subcutaneous insulin

Simulation Checklist		Time	Comments
Initial response	Recognition of diabetic ketoacidosis		
	Priority given to fluid resuscitation while awaiting lab confirmation		
IV fluids	Initial therapy with normal saline 1 L/hour × 2 hours		
	After first 2 L, IV fluids decreased to 250–500 mL/hour		
	Change to 1/2NS if corrected Na+ >140		
Potassium	Check potassium prior to giving insulin		
	Because K+ is 3.3–5.2, add 20 mEq/L of K+ to IV fluids		
Glucose	Give 8–10 unit bolus of insulin		
	Begin IV insulin drip at 0.1 unit/kg/hour		
	Add D5 to IV fluids when glucose <250		
pH	Because pH > 7.0, no bicarbonate necessary		
Fetal monitoring	Initiate fetal monitoring when maternal status is stable enough to consider cesarean		
	Treat maternal status to resuscitate signs of fetal acidemia		

Technical Skills	Non-Technical Skills
List risk factors for diabetic ketoacidosis	Use direct communication
List laboratory findings in diabetic ketoacidosis	Prioritize maternal resuscitation during acidosis
Describe management plan for patient with diabetic ketoacidosis	Communicate with patient

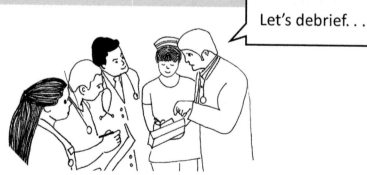

Let's debrief. . .

Technical and nontechnical skills for management of diabetic ketoacidosis.

Thyroid Storm

Thyroid storm and thyrotoxic heart failure are life-threatening hypermetabolic states in pregnancy. Thermoregulation, cardiovascular, nervous, and gastrointestinal systems can be affected, typically leading to multisystem failure (Fig. 23.1). The key to management is to have a high index of suspicion.

PRECIPITATING FACTORS[1]

- Labor and delivery
- Surgery
- Trauma
- Preeclampsia
- Anemia
- Sepsis

DIAGNOSIS[1]

Signs and symptoms of thyroid storm are frequently nonspecific. They include the following:

- Hyperthermia
- Nausea

| Tachycardia Congestive heart failure Arrhythmia | Agitation Confusion | Abdominal pain Nausea, vomiting | Hyperthermia Diaphoresis Dehydration |

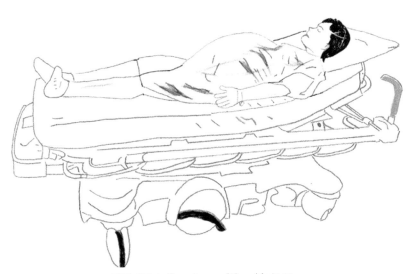

FIG. 23.1 Symptoms of thyroid storm.

Safety Training for Obstetric Emergencies. https://doi.org/10.1016/B978-0-323-69672-2.00023-0

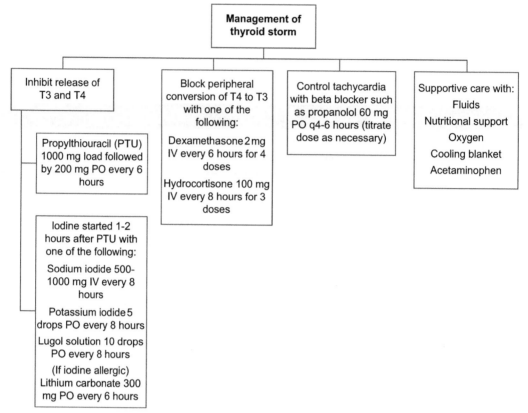

FIG. 23.2 Management of thyroid storm.

- Abdominal pain
- Vomiting
- Agitation
- Diaphoresis
- Dehydration
- Tachycardia
- Congestive heart failure
- Arrhythmia
- Confusion
- Cardiovascular collapse
- Malignant exophthalmos

The diagnosis is confirmed by low TSH and elevated T4.

MANAGEMENT[1,2]

Therapy should be initiated promptly once the diagnosis is suspected, even if thyroid tests are not back. An approach to management is outlined in Fig. 23.2.

REFERENCES

1. Waltman PA, Brewer JM, Lobert S. Thyroid storm during pregnancy. A medical emergency. *Crit Care Nurse*. 2004; 24(2):74–79.
2. American College of Obstetricians and Gynecologists. Practice bulletin No. 148: thyroid disease in pregnancy. *Obstet Gynecol*. 2015;125(4):996–1005.

Thyroid Storm Simulation

MATERIALS NEEDED
- Volunteer to act as standardized patient

KEY PERSONNEL
- Attending obstetrician
- Resident physician (if available in your institution)
- Nurse

SAMPLE SCENARIO
A 34-year-old G2P1 female at 32 weeks gestation presents with fever, vomiting, and "feeling like [her] heart is racing." On exam, her pulse is 154. BP is 176/98. Temperature is 104.1. She appears agitated. You note marked exophthalmos. Fetal heart rate tracing shows baseline of 180 with minimal variability, no accelerations, and no decelerations.

- Discuss your differential diagnosis. What would be your initial work-up and management for this patient?

- As you are waiting for other lab results, her TSH results as <0.01. How do you continue to manage this patient?

DEBRIEFING AND DOCUMENTATION
- Suspected precipitating factor for thyroid storm
- Medications received
- Fluids received
- Current vital signs
- Fetal status

Simulation Checklist

		Time	Comments
Recognition of thyroid storm	Considered thyroid storm on differential diagnosis		
	Initiated supportive measures without waiting for confirmation of diagnosis		
	Considered causes for thyroid storm		
Inhibit release of T3 and T4	PTU 1000 mg load followed by 200 mg every 6 hours		
	Iodine administration: • Sodium iodide 500–1000 mg IV every 8 hours *or* • Potassium iodide 5 drops PO every 8 hours *or* • Lugol solution 10 drops PO every 8 hours *or* • (if iodine allergic) Lithium carbonate 300 mg PO every 6 hours		
Block peripheral conversion of T4 to T3	Steroid administration: • Dexamethasone 2 mg IV every 6 hours for 4 doses *or* • Hydrocortisone 100 mg IV every 8 hours for 3 doses		
Control tachycardia	Beta blocker administration		
Supportive care	IV fluids		
	Oxygen		
	Cooling blanket		
	Acetaminophen		

Technical Skills	Non-Technical Skills
List risk factors for thyroid storm	Use direct communication
List laboratory findings in thyroid storm	Prioritize maternal resuscitation during thyroid storm
Describe management plan for patient with thyroid storm	Communicate with patient

Technical and nontechnical skills for management of thyroid storm.

Pheochromocytoma in Pregnancy

Pheochromocytoma is a catecholamine-secreting tumor that arises from chromaffin cells of the adrenal medulla or the sympathetic ganglia.

CLINICAL PRESENTATION[1]

- Symptoms (Fig. 24.1):
  - Severe hypertension—often difficult to control. Patient may have paradoxical supine hypertension with normal blood pressure in the sitting or erect position. This is because the gravid uterus can compress the tumor in the supine position and trigger catecholamine release
  - Paroxysmal or persistent hypertension
  - Headaches
  - Palpitations
  - Sweating
  - Panic attack-type symptoms
- Presents similarly to hypertensive disorders of pregnancy, but pheochromocytoma rarely has proteinuria and in pheochromocytoma the hypertension persists after childbirth (Table 24.1)

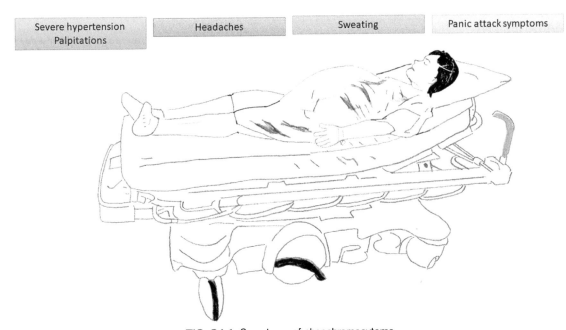

| Severe hypertension Palpitations | Headaches | Sweating | Panic attack symptoms |

FIG. 24.1 Symptoms of pheochromocytoma.

Safety Training for Obstetric Emergencies. https://doi.org/10.1016/B978-0-323-69672-2.00024-2

DIAGNOSIS

- Initial diagnosis is made by measurement of blood and/or urine catecholamines and their metabolites. As in nonpregnant women, the diagnosis is usually based upon the results of 24-hour urinary fractionated metanephrines and catecholamines and plasma fractionated metanephrines. However, clinicians must be aware that treatment with labetalol may give false positive results to this test[2]
- The localization of the neoplasm includes the use of ultrasound, MRI, and CT scan[3]
  - MRI examination (without gadolinium) has high sensitivity and specificity in pregnancy
  - Ultrasound is convenient with no harm to the fetus and is often the first method to discover pheochromocytoma during pregnancy. The disadvantage is poor sensitivity, especially for small adrenal pheochromocytomas and extra-adrenal paragangliomas
  - CT scan examination has a high sensitivity for the diagnosis of pheochromocytoma. However, its use in pregnancy is limited due to concerns for fetal exposure to radiation
  - Nuclear examination such as 131I iodo benzyl guanidine (MIBG) scintigraphy and octreotide are specific and sensitive diagnostic methods but are not appropriate during pregnancy

MANAGEMENT

Fig. 24.2 describes the management of pheochromocytoma in pregnancy. However it is important to emphasize that optimal management of pheochromocytoma in pregnancy is unclear. Treatment of pheochromocytoma during pregnancy should be based on different physiological characteristics and functional status of pheochromocytoma. Surgery is advocated by some authors if the fetus is previable (less than 24 weeks of gestation) and medical management when the pregnancy is further along. The rationale for surgery is that phenoxybenzamine crosses the placenta, and reports of perinatal depression and transient hypotension have been described. Other authors suggest that mid-pregnancy is an ideal time for surgery, because of the relatively low incidence of spontaneous abortion. In this period, the fetal organ development has been basically completed, and the uterine size has less impact on surgery.[3]

Medical Management

- Medical therapy should be initiated with α-adrenergic blockade (usually phenoxybenzamine)
- If necessary, this can be followed by β-adrenergic blockade

Surgical Management[4]

- Patients should be stabilited before going to the operating room
- Laparoscopic tumor resection during pregnancy appears to be safe and effective
- Advantages of laparoscopic resection include the following:
  - Reduced surgical trauma
  - Reduced blood loss
  - Decreased postoperative analgesia requirements
  - Avoids excessive compression of tumors and therefore intraoperative hemodynamic fluctuations
- Concerns regarding laparoscopic resection during pregnancy include the following:
  - The pneumoperitoneum might affect the blood supply of uterus
  - Increased abdominal pressure may trigger preterm labor
  - Increased abdominal pressure could induce hypertension
  - Hypercapnia could cause fetal acidosis
  - Pneumoperitoneum could cause fetal hypoxia by decreased cardiac output

Delivery Considerations

Spontaneous labor and delivery should be avoided. Cesarean delivery appears to carry less risk of maternal death than vaginal delivery.

TABLE 24.1 When to Suspect Pheochromocytoma in a Pregnant Patient
Intermittent labile blood pressures
Alternating hyper- and hypotension
Hypertension that worsens with beta-blockers
Paroxysmal symptoms of anxiety, diaphoresis, headache, palpitations, etc.
Family history of pheochromocytoma
Café-au-lait macules

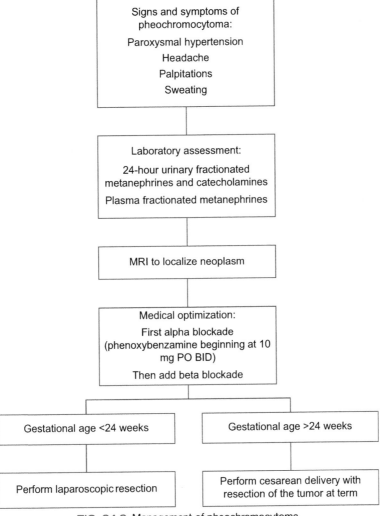

FIG. 24.2 Management of pheochromocytoma.

REFERENCES

1. Dong D, Li H. Diagnosis and treatment of pheochromocytoma during pregnancy. *J Matern Fetal Neonatal Med.* 2014;27(18):1930–1934.
2. Feldman JM. Falsely elevated urinary excretion of catecholamines and metanephrines in patients receiving labetalol therapy. *J Clin Pharmacol.* 1987;27(4):288–292.
3. van der Weerd K, et al. ENDOCRINOLOGY IN PREGNANCY: pheochromocytoma in pregnancy: case series and review of literature. *Eur J Endocrinol.* 2017;177(2): R49–R58.
4. FA EP, et al. Laparoscopic approach to pheochromocytoma in pregnancy: case report. *Int Braz J Urol.* 2018;44(3): 629–633.

Pheochromocytoma Simulation

MATERIALS NEEDED
- Volunteer to act as standardize patient

KEY PERSONNEL
- Attending obstetrician
- Resident physician (if available in your institution)
- Nurse

SAMPLE SCENARIO
A 36-year-old G1P0 female at 18 weeks gestation presents with episodes of headache, sweating, and palpitations. Her blood pressure during one of these episodes is recorded as 186/102.
   Discuss your differential diagnosis. How would you work up this patient?
   However, when you arrive the blood pressure is 90/50. Describe your management for this patient.

DEBRIEFING AND DOCUMENTATION
- How was diagnosis made
- Treatment sequence
- Clinical outcome
- Follow-up needed

Simulation Checklist

		Time	Comments
Differential diagnosis	Preeclampsia		
	Pheochromocytoma		
	Panic attacks		
	Drug abuse		
	Chronic hypertension		
Work-up	Urine protein		
	Urine drug screen		
	Urinary fractionated metanephrines and catecholamines		
	Complete blood cell count		
	Complete metabolic panel		
	Plasma fractionated metanephrines		
	After bloodwork supports pheochromocytoma, MRI		
Management	Initiation of α-blockade (phenoxybenzamine)		
	β-blockade only after α-blockade		
	Laparoscopic resection		

Technical Skills	Non-Technical Skills
List clinical signs of pheochromocytoma	Use direct communication
List laboratory findings in pheochromocytoma	Involve interdisciplinary team
Describe management plan for patient with pheochromocytoma	Communicate with patient

Technical and nontechnical skills for management of pheochromocytoma.

Amniotic Fluid Embolism

Amniotic fluid embolism is a fortunately rare obstetric emergency. However, if mothers are to survive this catastrophic event, clinicians must recognize it quickly and manage it very aggressively.

PATHOPHYSIOLOGY

Amniotic fluid embolism occurs when there is enhanced communication between the amniotic cavity and maternal circulation. This allows amniotic fluid to enter the maternal circulation where it triggers a systemic inflammatory response (Fig. 25.1). In the first hour, this typically presents as pulmonary hypertension and right ventricular failure. This is followed by left ventricular failure. The resultant hypotension and hypoxemia trigger multisystem organ failure. Concurrent activation of the coagulation cascade results in disseminated intravascular coagulation.[1,2]

Hypotension Right ventricular failure Left ventricular failure Cardiac arrhythmia Cardiac arrest	Proinflammatory state Disseminated intravascular coagulation Hemorrhage	Unexplained respiratory distress Dyspnea Hypoxemia	Fetal bradycardia
			Multisystem organ failure

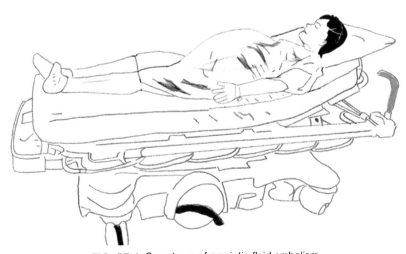

FIG. 25.1 Symptoms of amniotic fluid embolism.

Safety Training for Obstetric Emergencies. https://doi.org/10.1016/B978-0-323-69672-2.00025-4

TABLE 25.1
Management of Amniotic Fluid Embolism[1,2]

Cardiovascular	• Goal MAP is >65 mm Hg
	• Treat hypotension with vasopressors
	  - Norepinephrine 0.05-3.3 µg/kg/min
	  - Dobutamine 2.5-5.0 µg/kg/min
	• Avoid excessive fluid administration
	• If cardiac arrest, follow ACLS algorithms
	• Institute post-arrest hypothermia only if there is no clinical evidence of coagulopathy

Respiratory	• Supplemental oxygen should be titrated to maintain SpO$_2$ at 94–98% • Avoid hyperoxia after cardiac arrest (may worsen ischemia-reperfusion injury) • Intubation is commonly needed
Coagulopathy	• Aggressive blood replacement (including red blood cells, fresh frozen plasma, cryoprecipitate, and platelets) is critical • Consider activating massive transfusion protocol • Replacement can be initiated before clinical evidence of coagulopathy
Delivery	• If vaginal delivery is imminent, can proceed with assisted second stage • If not, proceed with immediate cesarean

RISK FACTORS[2,3]

- Multifetal gestation
- Advanced maternal age
- Operative delivery
- Eclampsia
- Polyhydramnios
- Cervical laceration
- Uterine rupture
- Placenta previa
- Amnioinfusion

CLINICAL PRESENTATION[1,2]

There are no diagnostic tests or laboratory findings for amniotic fluid embolism. It is a clinical diagnosis based on the following findings:

- Sudden, unexplained respiratory distress
- Hypotension
- Cardiac arrest
- Seizure-like activity
- Fetal bradycardia
- Disseminated intravascular coagulation
- Uterine atony

DIFFERENTIAL DIAGNOSIS

- Pulmonary embolism
- Congestive heart failure
- Myocardial infarction
- Anaphylaxis
- Placental abruption
- Sepsis with hypotension
- Placental abruption
- Anesthetic complications

MANAGEMENT[1,2]

The goals of management are stabilization of the mother and rapid delivery of the fetus (Table 25.1).

REFERENCES

1. Clark SL. Amniotic fluid embolism. *Obstet Gynecol.* 2014; 123(2 Pt 1):337–348.
2. Society for Maternal-Fetal Medicine, Electronic address, p.s.o, et al. Amniotic fluid embolism: diagnosis and management. *Am J Obstet Gynecol.* 2016;215(2):B16–B24.
3. Fong A, et al. Amniotic fluid embolism: antepartum, intrapartum and demographic factors. *J Matern Fetal Neonatal Med.* 2015;28(7):793–798.

Amniotic Fluid Embolism Simulation

MATERIALS NEEDED
- Manikin
- Laryngoscope
- Endotracheal tube
- Adult code cart

KEY PERSONNEL
- Anesthesiologist
- Attending obstetrician
- Neonatologist
- Resident physician (if available in your institution)
- Two nurses

SAMPLE SCENARIO

A 42-year-old G3P2 female at 37 weeks gestation is admitted in active labor. Patient's pregnancy has been uncomplicated other than idiopathic polyhydramnios. On admission, her cervix is 6 cm dilated. Fetal heart tracing is 135 beats per minute with moderate variability, accelerations, and no decelerations. She is contracting every 5 minutes.

Shortly after admission, the patient experiences spontaneous rupture of membranes. She becomes agitated and begins to complain that she cannot breathe. Her respiratory rate climbs to 26 breaths per minute. A pulse oximeter reveals an oxygen saturation of 74%. The patient's blood pressure is 84/44 mm Hg and pulse is 145 beats per minute. The fetal heart rate is now 100 beats per minute.

DEBRIEFING AND DOCUMENTATION
- Diagnosis and how it was made
- If cardiac arrest occurred, document thoroughly resuscitation
- Respiratory interventions-current ventilator settings
- Delivery information
  - Time for decision-to-delivery
  - Mode of delivery
  - Infant status
  - Blood loss
- If postpartum hemorrhage occurred, document interventions
- Blood products given
- Labs ordered
- Imaging ordered
- Consultants contacted
- Communication with patient and family

Simulation Checklist

		Time	Comments
Initial response	Recognized emergency		
	Called for help		
Team dynamics	Team leader identified		
	Team member roles clearly assigned		
	Considered differential diagnoses		
Circulation	Applied blood pressure cuff, cardiac monitor		
	Avoided excessive fluid administration		
	Identified goal MAP of >65 mm Hg		
	Treated of hypotension with vasopressors		
	Confirm adult code cart is readily available		
	EKG ordered		
Airway and breathing	Lungs auscultated		
	Supplemental oxygen given		
	FiO_2 titrated to keep SpO_2 94%–98%		
	Considered need for intubation		
	Pulse ox requested		
	ABG ordered		
Pregnancy-related considerations	IV access obtained above diaphragm		
	Left uterine displacement		
	Decision made to proceed with cesarean		
	Prepared for postpartum hemorrhage		
Coagulopathy	Considered likelihood of coagulopathy if amniotic fluid embolism		
	Prepared for massive transfusion		
Documentation	Persons present		
	Maternal vitals		
	Fetal/neonatal status		
	Interventions		
	Timing of delivery		
	Differential diagnosis		
	Management plan		
Communication	Succinctly summarized situation, background, assessment, and recommendations as help arrived		
	Directed communication		
	Closed-loop communication		
	Communication with patient and family		

Technical Skills	Non-Technical Skills
Provide supplemental oxygen	Communication with team members
Perform intubation	Situational awareness
Perform ACLS resuscitation	Debrief with team
Perform immediate delivery	Communicate with patient and family

Let's debrief. . .

Technical and nontechnical skills in management of amniotic fluid embolism.

Myasthenia Gravis

PATHOPHYSIOLOGY[1,2]

- Autoimmune disease resulting from antibodies against the acetylcholine receptor or muscle-specific kinase
- When antibodies bind to acetylcholine receptor, it blocks muscle contraction and results in weakness of skeletal muscles
- Antibodies frequently result from the presence of a thymoma

SIGNS AND SYMPTOMS[1]

- Fatigable, painless muscle weakness
- Double vision and ptosis (Fig. 26.1) are common
- Often difficulty with chewing, swallowing

DIAGNOSIS[1,3]

- Edrophonium (Tensilon) test
  - Edrophonium is used because it is a short-acting anticholinesterase medication
  - To perform test, 0.5-1.0 mg of edrophonium is given[4]
  - The patient is observed for clinical resolution of ptosis occurring within 30-60 seconds of the medication
- Serum autoantibody analysis
- Electromyography shows rapid decline in size of evoked muscle action potentials

TREATMENT[1,4-6]

- Acetylcholinesterase inhibitors—decrease acetylcholine destruction at neuromuscular junction
  - Pyridostigmine—first-line treatment in pregnancy (60 mg every 4–6 hours)
  - Neostigmine (15 mg every 2–3 hours)

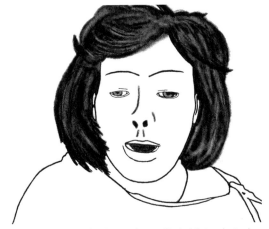

FIG. 26.1 Myasthenia gravis results in bilateral ptosis.

- Immunosuppressive medications
  - Corticosteroids—preferred immunosuppressive during pregnancy
  - Azathioprine (2–3 mg/kg/day)
  - Calcineurin
- Intravenous immunoglobulin (IVIG) and plasma exchange—used in patients with acute exacerbation for rapid but temporary stabilization
- Thymectomy is deferred until postpartum

DELIVERY CONSIDERATIONS[2,5,7]

- Patient's medications should be continued during labor and delivery
- Vaginal delivery preferred
- Assisted second stage of labor may be necessary
- Magnesium sulfate is contraindicated
- If antihypertensives are needed, preferred agents are methyldopa or hydralazine

Safety Training for Obstetric Emergencies. https://doi.org/10.1016/B978-0-323-69672-2.00026-6

ANESTHESIA CONCERNS[1,8-9]

- Early neuraxial anesthesia protects from overexertion, fatigue
  - Amide-type medications are acceptable
  - Ester-type medications can exacerbate myasthenia
- If general anesthesia is required, avoid muscle relaxants and succinylcholine
  - Volatile anesthetics are preferred
  - Train-of-four "twitch" monitoring is used to assess degree of neuromuscular blockade
  - Do NOT extubate until twitch monitoring shows reversal of blockade
- Sedatives and opioids should be used with caution as they can worsen respiratory status

MYASTHENIC CRISIS[2]

- When respiratory muscles are affected to the degree that the patient is unable to ventilate appropriately
- Requires mechanical ventilation

NEONATAL CONCERNS[2,10-11]

- Neonatal effects not well correlated with maternal disease severity
- In 10%–20% of pregnancies, transplacental passage of antibodies can cause myasthenic symptoms in neonate
- Symptoms include difficulty breathing and feeding
- All neonates should be observed for 48–72 hours for signs of neonatal myasthenia
- Affected infants can be managed with pyridostigmine and ventilator support

REFERENCES

1. Varner M. Myasthenia gravis and pregnancy. *Clin Obstet Gynecol.* 2013;56(2):372–381.
2. Roth CK, Dent S, McDevitt K. Myasthenia gravis in pregnancy. *Nurs Womens Health.* 2015;19(3):248–252.
3. Pascuzzi RM. The edrophonium test. *Semin Neurol.* 2003; 21(1):83–88.
4. Norwood F, et al. Myasthenia in pregnancy: best practice guidelines from a U.K. multispecialty working group. *J Neurol Neurosurg Psychiatry.* 2014;85(5):538–543.
5. Sanders DB, et al. International consensus guidance for management of myasthenia gravis: executive summary. *Neurology.* 2016;87(4):419–425.
6. Gamez J, et al. Intravenous immunoglobulin as monotherapy for myasthenia gravis during pregnancy. *J Neurol Sci.* 2017;383:118–122.
7. Massey JM, De Jesus-Acosta C. Pregnancy and myasthenia gravis. *Continuum (Minneap Minn).* 2014;20(1 Neurology of Pregnancy):115–127.
8. Hopkins AN, et al. Neurologic disease with pregnancy and considerations for the obstetric anesthesiologist. *Semin Perinatol.* 2014;38(6):359–369.
9. Tsurane K, Tanabe S, Miyasaka N, Matsuda M, Takahara M, Ida T, Kohyama A. Management of labor and delivery in myasthenia gravis: a new protocol. *J Obstet Gynaecol Res;* 2019. E-pub https://doi.org/10.1111/jog.13922.
10. Jovandaric MZ, et al. Neonatal outcome in pregnancies with autoimmune myasthenia gravis. *Fetal Pediatr Pathol.* 2016;35(3):167–172.
11. Ducci RD, et al. Clinical follow-up of pregnancy in myasthenia gravis patients. *Neuromuscul Disord.* 2017;27(4): 352–357.

Myasthenia Gravis Simulation

MATERIALS NEEDED
- Manikin or volunteer to act as standardized patient

KEY PERSONNEL
- Anesthesiologist
- Attending obstetrician
- Nurse
- Resident physician (if available in your institution)

SAMPLE SCENARIO
A 26-year-old G2P1 with history of myasthenia gravis presents in labor. She progresses to fully dilated. Shortly after she begins pushing, she complains of shortness of breath. Her SpO$_2$ is 89%. The patient is notable taking shallow breaths. How do you proceed?

DEBRIEFING AND DOCUMENTATION
- When was respiratory distress noted?
- Interventions initiated for maternal respiratory status
- How delivery accomplished
- Description of maternal and/or neonatal injuries
- Communication with family

Simulation Checklist

		Time	Comments
Recognize	Recognized maternal respiratory distress		
	Recognized risk factors in clinical history		
Call for help	Summoned appropriate help urgently		
	Called for experienced help, especially anesthesiologist		
Airway, breathing	Intubation performed		
	Mechanical ventilation initiated		
Delivery	Assisted second stage performed		
Documentation	Timing of events		
	Persons present		
Communication	Directed communication		
	Closed-loop communication		

Technical Skills	Non-Technical Skills
List medications used in myasthenia gravis	Communication with team members about diagnosis and precautions
Assessment of muscle function in patients with myasthenia gravis	Awareness of patient's respiratory status
Resuscitate neonate with congenital myasthenia	

Technical and nontechnical skills for management of myasthenia gravis.

Autonomic Dysreflexia

PATHOPHYSIOLOGY[1–3]

- Occurs in 85% of women with spinal cord injury at level of T6 or above
- When the woman experiences a painful stimulus below the level of the spinal injury (such as from contractions or even a full bladder), she may not be conscious of the pain but it is still perceived by the sympathetic nerve fibers
- Because the sympathetic nerve fibers in the spinal cord are separated from their normal inhibition from the brain, the painful stimulus results in a hypersympathetic response (Fig. 27.1)
- This hypersympathetic response results in dangerously elevated blood pressure, cardiac arrhythmias, and other symptoms (Fig. 27.2)

SIGNS AND SYMPTOMS[1–4]

- Severe hypertension
- Cardiac arrhythmia (bradycardia, atrial fibrillation, premature ventricular contractions, conduction abnormalities)
- Hyperthermia
- Sweating

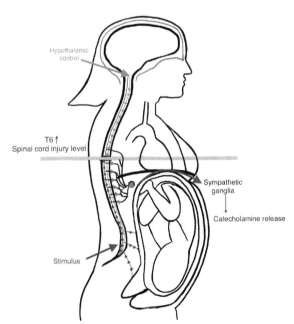

FIG. 27.1 Spinal cord injury prevents descending regulation of efferent sympathetic spinal neurons. Therefore, noxious stimuli result in a reflexic hypersympathetic response.

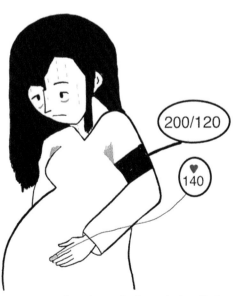

FIG. 27.2 Symptoms of autonomic dysreflexia.

Safety Training for Obstetric Emergencies. https://doi.org/10.1016/B978-0-323-69672-2.00027-8

- Flushing
- Dilated pupils
- Increased spasticity
- Seizures
- Stroke
- Coma
- Death

MANAGEMENT[1,2,5,6]

- Remove noxious stimulus
  - If the bladder is distended → drain it
  - If clothing is too tight → loosen it
  - If the stimulus is labor pain → initiate epidural early in labor and continue for 24–48 hours postpartum
- Elevate the head of the bed
- Monitor BP every 2–5 minutes until patient stabilized
- If systolic blood pressure is sustained >150 mmHg, give 10 mg sublingual nifedipine

REFERENCES

1. Camune BD. Challenges in the management of the pregnant woman with spinal cord injury. *J Perinat Neonatal Nurs.* 2013;27(3):225–231.
2. Gunduz H, Binak DF. Autonomic dysreflexia: an important cardiovascular complication in spinal cord injury patients. *Cardiol J.* 2012;19(2):215–219.
3. Pope CS, Markenson GR, Bayer-Zwirello LA, et al. Pregnancy complicated by chronic spinal cord injury and history of autonomic hyperreflexia. *Obstet Gynecol.* 2001;97(5 Pt 2): 802–803.
4. Castro JS, Lourenco C, Carrilho M. Successful pregnancy in a woman with paraplegia. *BMJ Case Rep.* 2014;2014.
5. Krassioukov A, Warburton DE, Teasell R, et al. A systematic review of the management of autonomic dysreflexia after spinal cord injury. *Arch Phys Med Rehabil.* 2009;90(4): 682–695.
6. Le Liepvre H, Dinh A, Idiard-Chamois B, et al. Pregnancy in spinal cord-injured women, a cohort study of 37 pregnancies in 25 women. *Spinal Cord.* 2017;55(2): 167–171.

Autonomic Dysreflexia Simulation

MATERIALS NEEDED
- Manikin or person to act as patient

KEY PERSONNEL
- Anesthesiologist
- Attending obstetrician
- Nurse
- Resident physician (if available in your institution)

SAMPLE SCENARIO
Maria is a 25-year-old G1P0 at 38 weeks 4 days gestation who presents with leaking fluid. She has a history of spinal cord injury at T5 following a motor vehicle accident 13 months ago. As a result, patient has lack of sensation or strength in her legs, abdomen, and torso. While she is being evaluated, she complains of a throbbing headache. Her blood pressure is 220/115. You note sweating and increased spasticity.

DEBRIEFING AND DOCUMENTATION
- Recognition of autonomic dysreflexia
- Differential diagnosis
- Measures to limit noxious stimuli
- Measures to stabilize maternal blood pressure
- Communication with patient and family

Simulation Checklist

		Time	Comments
Initial response	Recognized signs of autonomic dysreflexia		
	Called for help		
	Raised head of bed		
Address noxious stimulus	Checked for distended bladder		
	Checked for fecal impaction		
	Provided adequate labor pain relief		
	Loosened tight clothing		
Address blood pressure	Monitored blood pressure every 2–5 minutes		
	Treated persistently elevated blood pressure with nifedipine 10 mg sublingual		
Documentation	Time of symptom onset		
	Interventions		
	Vital signs		
	Time of maternal stabilization		
Communication	Kept patient and partner informed		
	Directed communication		
	Closed-loop communication		

Technical Skills	Non-Technical Skills
Knowledge of management of pathophysiology of autonomic dysreflexia	Communication with team members about risk of autonomic dysrelfexia
Knowledge of management algorithms for autonomic dysreflexia	Awareness of signs and symptoms of autonomic dysreflexia
Placement of epidural anesthesia	Task management

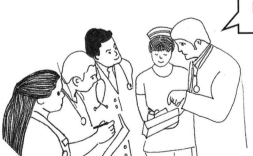

Let's debrief. . .

Technical and nontechnical skills for autonomic dysreflexia.

CHAPTER 28

Trauma in Pregnancy

LEARNING OBJECTIVES

- Describe the basic principles of trauma management in pregnancy.
- Demonstrate how to triage trauma patients to guide management.
- List signs of trauma-related placental abruption.

Trauma in pregnancy is the main cause of maternal death due to nonobstetrical etiologies.[1] Trauma-associated placental abruption is a major contributor to perinatal death.[2,3]

COMMON CAUSES OF TRAUMA IN PREGNANCY[4]

- Domestic violence
- Motor vehicle crashes
- Falls
- Homicide
- Suicide

OBSTETRICAL COMPLICATIONS OF TRAUMA[3]

- Preterm labor
- Premature rupture of membranes
- Uterine rupture
- Spontaneous abortion
- Intrauterine fetal demise

DEFINING TRAUMA SEVERITY

The severity of trauma is directly related to maternal and fetal outcomes. However, because minor trauma is more common, 60%–70% of fetal losses are due to minor trauma.[2]

Defining features of "major trauma" are as follows:[2,5]

- Unstable vital signs
- Altered consciousness
- Trauma involving the abdomen

- Rapid compression, deceleration, or shearing forces
- Trauma that results in vaginal bleeding, abdominal pain, and/or decreased fetal movements
- Trauma that results in more than minor bruising, lacerations, or contusions

GENERAL PRINCIPLES OF TRAUMA MANAGEMENT IN PREGNANCY

- Maintain a multidisciplinary approach and good communication among team members
- Every healthcare facility should be prepared for initial evaluation, stabilization, and care of the pregnant patient
- Transportation to the ideal trauma care center should be considered depending on risk–benefit ratio and the specific trauma circumstances
- Maternal health is the primary goal in the management of trauma in pregnancy. Interventions for fetal benefit should be only carried out after stabilization of the mother
- Advanced trauma life support (ATLS) and advanced cardiac life support (ACLS) guidelines should be followed
- Perimortem cesarean delivery should be performed for any pregnancies greater than 20 weeks if maternal cardiac arrest lasts for greater than 4 minutes. Do not delay delivery because of operating room transportation, abdomen sterilization, or confirmation of fetal viability
- No diagnostic or therapeutic interventions should be withheld because of the concern for potential undesired fetal effects

Safety Training for Obstetric Emergencies. https://doi.org/10.1016/B978-0-323-69672-2.00028-X

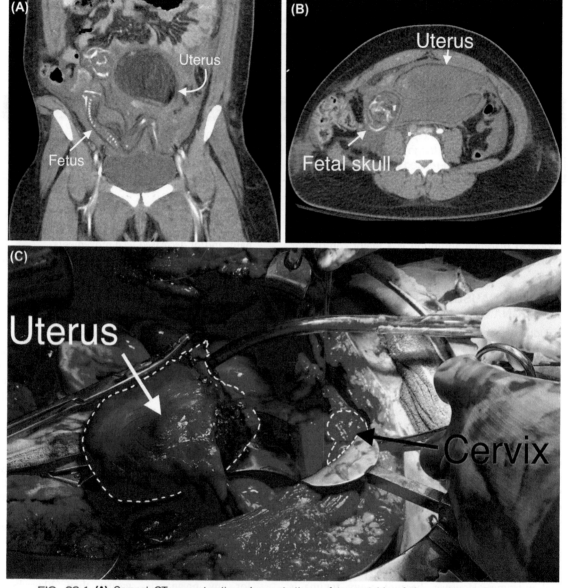

FIG. 28.1 **(A)** Coronal CT reconstruction, demonstrating a fetus outside of the uterine cavity and a "discontinuous uterus" suggesting uterine rupture. **(B)** Transverse CT demonstrates a fetus outside of the uterine cavity and a "discontinuous skull" suggesting fetal cranial injury. **(C)** Laparotomy, confirming uterine avulsion; The uterus and the cervix are separated, as consequence of the trauma. The fetus was in the abdomen at delivery.

- Imaging
  - Computed tomography (CT) scan may be useful in the diagnosis of placental abruption and/or uterine rupture.[6] Fig. 28.1 shows CT findings in a patient with complete uterine avulsion and fetal demise secondary to motor vehicle accident

- The typical CT scan radiation dose is not associated with adverse outcomes[7]
- Focused assessment with sonography for trauma (F.A.S.T) is an efficient method for detection of intraabdominal free fluid and organ injuries; it consists in the assessment of free fluid in four

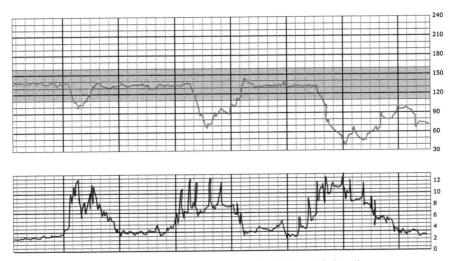

FIG. 28.2 Posttrauma NST suggestive of placental abruption.

areas: right and left upper quadrants, suprapubic, and subxiphoid areas[8]

- Hemorrhage control
  - Intracavitary hemorrhage may require activation of massive transfusion protocols. A suggested approach is a 1:1:1 replacement of fresh frozen plasma, platelets, and packed red blood cells
  - Cryoprecipitate and prothrombin complex concentrate may be necessary
  - Topical hemostatic agents are considered safe to use during pregnancy
  - Tranexamic acid use seems safe for the fetus but has an unclear effect on maternal mortality
- Sepsis is a risk for admitted patient with major trauma, burns, and penetrating injuries
- These fetal interventions can follow or be undertaken simultaneously with maternal stabilization:
  - Leftward uterine displacement
  - Volume replacement
  - Oxygen administration
  - Cesarean delivery

TRAUMA-RELATED PLACENTAL ABRUPTION

- Abruption is a clinical diagnosis
- Trauma patients may develop "concealed" abruption without vaginal bleeding
- Cardiotocography has a high negative predictive value for placental abruption[9]

- Continuous fetal monitoring allows timely identification of fetal distress that requires delivery (see Fig. 28.2)[10]

MANAGEMENT ALGORITHMS BASED ON TRAUMA SEVERITY

Management of maternal trauma begins with a primary survey and assessment of maternal stability as detailed in Fig. 28.3.

Management of a Hemodynamically Unstable and/or Unresponsive Mother

- Hemodynamic instability/unresponsiveness criteria
  - Blood pressure <80/40 mmHg
  - Pulse <50 or >140 beats per minute
  - Cardiac or respiratory arrest
  - Loss of airway
- Follow ACLS and ATLS guidelines
- If exploratory laparotomy is performed, it does not necessarily necessitate cesarean delivery
- Basic labs
  - Complete blood count
  - Chemistry panel
  - Type and cross
  - Kleihauer–Betke test (KB) if Rh negative
  - Coagulation profile
  - Toxicology screen

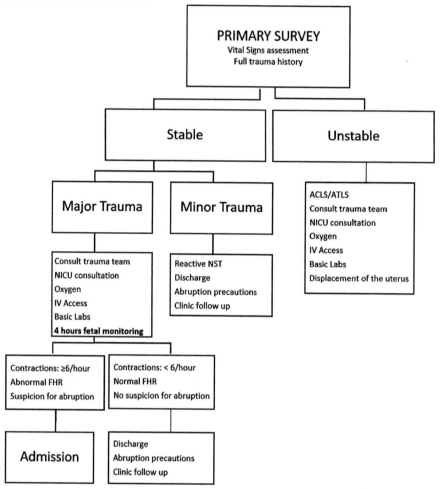

FIG. 28.3 Management of trauma in pregnancy based on maternal stability and trauma severity.

Management of a Hemodynamically Stable Mother With Major Trauma

- Administer Rh immunoglobulin within 72 hours if mother is Rh negative
- Perform a KB test for appropriate dosing of Rh immunoglobulin
- If fetus is viable
  - Perform continuous fetal monitoring for *at least* 4 hours
  - If patient is having fewer than six contractions per hour and no other concerns, discharge home with abruption precautions and clinical follow-up
  - If patient is having six or more contractions per hour, maintain continuous fetal monitoring for 24 hours

- If fetus is nonviable
  - Check the fetal heart rate with Doppler. If normal FHR and no other concerns, consider discharge home with abruption precautions and clinical follow-up
  - If there is concern for placental abruption, consider tocometry and admission for 24 hours monitoring

Management of a Hemodynamically Stable Mother With Minor Trauma

- If fetus is viable, perform a nonstress test (NST)
  - If NST is reactive and no further testing is recommended, discharge patient with abruption precautions and clinical follow-up[4]

- If NST is nonreactive, consider additional fetal well-being assessment and/or admission for monitoring
- If fetus is nonviable check fetal heart rate with Doppler.
  - If normal FHR and no other concerns, consider discharge with abruption precautions and clinical follow-up
  - If there is concern for placental abruption, consider tocometry and admission for 24 hours monitoring.

REFERENCES

1. Fildes J, Reed L, Jones N, Martin M, Barrett J. Trauma: the leading cause of maternal death. *J Trauma*. 1992;32: 643–645.
2. El-Kady D, Gilbert WM, Anderson J, Danielsen B, Towner D, Smith LH. Trauma during pregnancy: an analysis of maternal and fetal outcomes in a large population. *Am J Obstet Gynecol*. 2004;190: 1661–1668.
3. Shah KH, Simons RK, Holbrook T, Fortlage D, Winchell RJ, Hoyt DB. Trauma in pregnancy: maternal and fetal outcomes. *J Trauma*. 1998;45:83–86.
4. Mendez-Figueroa H, Dahlke JD, Vrees RA, Rouse DJ. Trauma in pregnancy: an updated systematic review. *Am J Obstet Gynecol*. 2013;209:1–10.
5. Cahill AG, Bastek JA, Stamilio DM, Odibo AO, Stevens E, Macones GA. Minor trauma in pregnancy–is the evaluation unwarranted? *Am J Obstet Gynecol*. 2008;198: 208 e1–5.
6. Jha P, Melendres G, Bijan B, et al. Trauma in pregnant women: assessing detection of post-traumatic placental abruption on contrast-enhanced CT versus ultrasound. *Abdom Radiol (NY)*. 2017;42:1062–1067.
7. Practice ACoO. ACOG Committee Opinion. Number 299, September 2004 (replaces No. 158, September 1995). Guidelines for diagnostic imaging during pregnancy. *Obstet Gynecol*. 2004;104:647–651.
8. Richards JR, Ormsby EL, Romo MV, Gillen MA, McGahan JP. Blunt abdominal injury in the pregnant patient: detection with US. *Radiology*. 2004;233: 463–470.
9. Connolly AM, Katz VL, Bash KL, McMahon MJ, Hansen WF. Trauma and pregnancy. *Am J Perinatol*. 1997;14:331–336.
10. Rogers FB, Rozycki GS, Osler TM, et al. A multi-institutional study of factors associated with fetal death in injured pregnant patients. *Arch Surg*. 1999;134: 1274–1277.

Trauma Simulation

MATERIALS NEEDED
- Manikin

KEY PERSONNEL
- Obstetrician
- Emergency room physician
- Anesthesiologist
- Neonatologist
- Resident physician (if available in your institution)
- Nurse

SAMPLE SCENARIO
A 28-year-old G1P0 at 32 weeks' gestation is brought in by Emergency Medical Services after being involved in a single-vehicle collision. Patient was a belted passenger. There is a bruise across her abdomen from the seatbelt. Patient is alert and conversant but complaining of abdominal pain.
- Her blood pressure is 105/78. Her pulse is 108. SpO2 is 98% on room air.
- Discuss evaluation and management of this patient.

DEBRIEFING AND DOCUMENTATION
- Steps taken for maternal stabilization
- Results of primary and secondary survey
- Description of fetal status
- Description of contractions
- Lab results
- Imaging results
- Plan for maternal and fetal surveillance

Simulation Checklist			Time	Comments
Primary survey	Assessed maternal airway			
	Assessed maternal breathing			
	Assessed for tissue perfusion (circulation)			
	Performed brief neurologic exam (disability)			
	Assessed for exposures (maintain normothermia)			
	Assessed of fetal heart rate			
Initial resuscitation	IV access obtained			
	IV fluid bolus given			
Laboratory tests	Complete blood count			
	Type and cross			
	Kleihauer–Betke test			
Fetal monitoring	Continuous fetal monitoring			
	Tocodynameter assessment			
Imaging studies	Consider CT scan, MRI, F.A.S. T			
Communication	Call-out			
	Directed communication			
	Closed-loop communication			

Technical Skills	Non-Technical Skills
List characteristics of major trauma	Prioritization of maternal resuscitation
Management algorithms	Communication with family
Nonstress test interpretation	Task management
Assessment of contractions	Teamwork

Let's debrief. . .

Pregnancies in Challenging Locations

There are times when a pregnancy implants in abnormal locations and develops to an advanced gestational age. Under certain circumstances, these pregnancies can result in delivery of a healthy infant. However, the safety of both the mother and the infant relies heavily on preoperative planning and an interdisciplinary approach. In this chapter, we review important considerations for interdisciplinary planning of these difficult cases. We report complex cases managed at our institution that resulted in positive outcomes for both the mother and the fetus.

INTERDISCIPLINARY PLANNING FOR COMPLEX SURGICAL CASES

Preoperative discussion should include representatives from many specialties, which depending on the clinical scenario may include the following steps:

- Obstetrics and Gynecology
- Maternal−fetal medicine
- Anesthesia
- General surgery
- Vascular surgery
- Urology
- Critical care
- Interventional radiology
- Neonatology
- Nursing

Topics to Discuss

- Timing of delivery (and if premature, should betamethasone and magnesium sulfate be administered?)

- Location of delivery
  - Is your institution appropriate for maternal and neonatal needs? If not, consider referral to tertiary care center
  - Within your institution, is patient better served in main operating room or labor and delivery unit?
- Preoperative imaging needed
- Preferred vascular access
- Anticipated operative approach
- Anticipated blood product needs
- Special equipment needs
- Anticipated postoperative needs

Communication With Patient and Family

- It is important to have an open and honest discussion with patient and her family about the risks to both her and the baby of the given condition
- Allow multiple opportunities for patient and family to ask questions, as their understanding of the condition will likely evolve over time
- On the day of the surgery, designate someone to keep the patient's family updated so the surgical team can focus on their primary responsibilities in the operating room

ABDOMINAL PREGNANCY

A patient presented to our institution at 27 weeks gestation because of a suspicion for an abnormal pregnancy. On ultrasound, the fetus was noted to be developing outside of the uterine cavity (Fig. 29.1A−D). Diagnosis of abdominal pregnancy was made. An interdisciplinary meeting was held that involved maternal−fetal

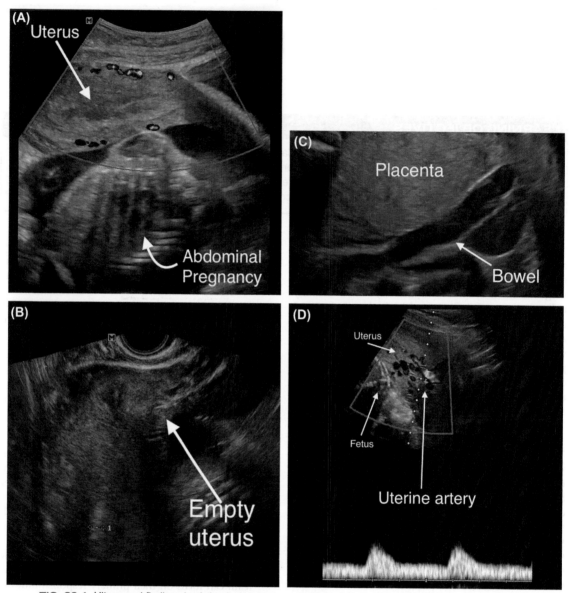

FIG. 29.1 Ultrasound findings in abdominal pregnancy at 27 weeks' gestation. **(A)** Note the fetus is behind the uterus. **(B)** Ultrasound of the uterus that is empty. **(C)** The placenta is implanted above the sigmoid colon. **(D)** Uterine artery with velocity waveforms; the uterine artery (red color) is directed towards the uterus.

medicine, vascular surgery, general surgery, anesthesia, and neonatology. Given the concern for unpredictable, catastrophic maternal hemorrhage, the decision was made to proceed with delivery after administration of antenatal steroids. At surgery, a midline incision was made. The gestational sac was noted to be intact, posterior to the uterus (Fig. 29.2). The membranes were ruptured, and the infant was delivered without difficulty. The vascular surgeon then identified and ligated

the maternal vessels that extended from the sigmoid colon to the placenta. The placenta was attached to the right adnexa, cul-de-sac, and sigmoid colon. The placenta was removed intact. Excellent hemostasis was obtained. Both the mother and the infant were discharged home in good condition.

A second case had occurred 5 years earlier at our institution. The pregnancy was at 35 weeks' gestation. There was no prenatal care. At cesarean delivery, the

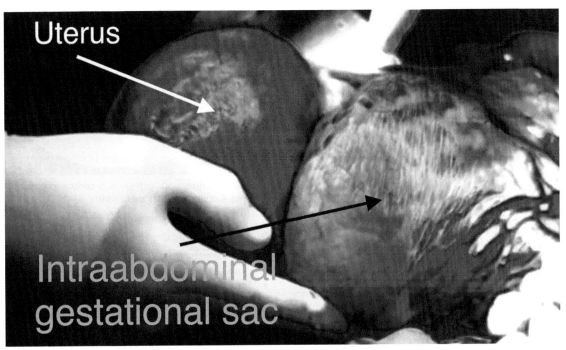

FIG. 29.2 Abdominal pregnancy with gestational sac behind the uterus.

placenta was found to be implanted on the omentum. It was removed and both mother and infant did well.

These two cases emphasize that an abdominal pregnancy may end with alive and healthy babies.

Clinical Signs of Healthy Abdominal Pregnancy[1]

- Inability to induce labor
- Abdominal pain, particularly with fetal movements
- Easy abdominal palpation of fetal parts

Ultrasound Findings in Abdominal Pregnancy

- Lack of myometrial wall between gestational sac and bladder[1]
- Suspected bicornuate uterus without myometrium surrounding the fetus[2]
- MRI can be useful to help clarify ultrasound findings[3]

Surgical Strategies for Abdominal Pregnancy

- Placenta can be successfully removed in majority of cases[1]
- Consult with vascular surgery to identify and ligate placental vessels before attempting placenta removal[1]
- If the placenta is attached to the uterus, a tourniquet can be applied to the lower uterine segment to reduce blood loss during uterine repair[4]

- A bleeding placental bed can often be controlled by placing abdominal packs and removing them after 48 hours[2,5]
- There are reports in the literature of leaving the placenta in situ and allowing for delayed resorption[6,7]; however, we believe that this can lead to recurrent maternal infections with risk of developing antimicrobial resistance. In the event of multidrug resistance, infection can be life-threatening

CESAREAN SCAR PREGNANCY

A cesarean scar pregnancy is suspected when the pregnancy appears implanted within the niche of the previous cesarean scar by ultrasound (Fig. 29.3). The optimal treatment is unknown. Termination of the pregnancy is an option. This can be either medical or surgical intervention. The following procedures have been reported in the literature: Systemic and local methotrexate, KCl, dilation and curettage, and wedge resection with laparoscopy or laparotomy.[8]

If the patient declines intervention, she is expectantly managed. These patients need to be followed for placental attachment pathology. We usually follow these patients with serial ultrasounds, and we deliver patients with accreta/increta/percreta between 34 and 36 weeks' gestation following steroids. When the

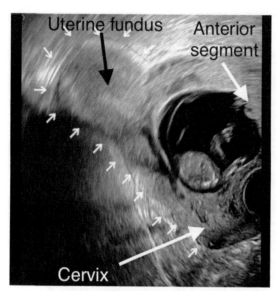

FIG. 29.3 Ultrasound findings in cesarean scar pregnancy at 11 weeks gestation.

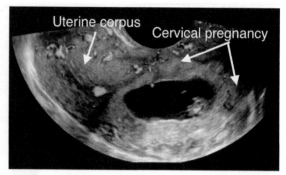

FIG. 29.4 Ultrasound findings in a cervical pregnancy at 7 weeks (Courtesy by Marcos Cordoba).

suspicion is high, following counseling of the patient, we perform a cesarean hysterectomy. For anesthesia, we usually use a combined spinal epidural anesthesia. The urologist places ureteral catheters. The interventional radiologist places but does not inflate internal iliac balloon catheters. A midline incision is usually made. A uterine incision that avoids the placenta is made. If the placenta is anterior we perform either a fundal incision or a posterior incision. After delivery, the uterus is closed with the placenta in situ, the iliac balloons are usually inflated, and a bilateral uterine artery ligation is performed. Next we proceed with the hysterectomy.

Ultrasound Findings in Cesarean Scar Pregnancy

- Gestational sac implanted within cesarean scar[9]
- Empty cervical canal[10]
- Thin myometrial layer between bladder and gestational sac[10]

Complications of Cesarean Scar Pregnancy Managed Expectantly

- Severe hemorrhage[11]
- Early uterine rupture[11]
- Placenta accreta spectrum[8,11,12]
- Hysterectomy[8,11]

Surgical Strategies for Advanced Cesarean Scar Pregnancy[13]

- Consider ureteral stents (unproven benefit)
- Consider iliac artery occlusion (unproven benefit)
- Plan skin incision that will allow good visualization and ability to make hysterotomy away from the placenta
- Do not attempt forced placental removal
- Consider use of tranexamic acid 1 g IV within 3 hours after birth; can be repeated once after 30 minutes if there is persistent bleeding

CERVICAL PREGNANCY

Definition

Cervical pregnancy is an ectopic pregnancy that has implanted in the endocervix.

The incidence is 1:14,000. Usually, it aborts in the first trimester but it can continue longer when it is implanted close to the uterine cavity.

Diagnosis

The most common sign is bleeding. The diagnosis is made by ultrasound. The ultrasound shows implantation at the cervical level with hypervascularity (Fig. 29.4).

Management

The treatments proposed are as follows:

- Methotrexate (systemic or local) with or without intraamniotic/intrafetal KCl.[14, 15]
- Tamponading with a Foley catheter or D&C + tamponading with a Foley catheter.[16]
- Embolization.[17]
- Hysterectomy

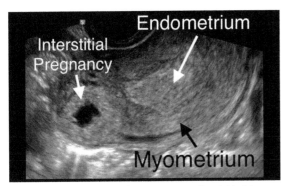

FIG. 29.5 Interstitial pregnancy on the right side.

When a cervical pregnancy is treated, it is important that the team is ready to perform a hysterectomy because the bleeding may be excessive and difficult to control.

The case in Fig. 29.4 was managed with intracervical Foley catheter alone. The patient did not require any other intervention.

Rarely, the pregnancy from the cervix grows inside the uterine cavity, and it may result in the birth of a live baby.

INTERSTITIAL PREGNANCY

An interstitial ectopic pregnancy occurs when the blastocyst implants in the interstitial portion of the fallopian tube as it enters the uterine cavity. Because it is surrounded by myometrium, the interstitial ectopic is often able to reach a larger size before becoming symptomatic. It is relatively rare, accounting for only 2%–4% of ectopic pregnancies.[18]

The diagnosis is made by ultrasound in combination with human chorionic gonadotropin. The ultrasound features that assist in the diagnosis of an interstitial ectopic are eccentric location in relation to the endometrial stripe, presence of myometrium surrounding most or all of the gestation (depending on size), and the interstitial line sign, which is an echogenic line extending from the gestational sac to the endometrium (Fig. 29.5).[19]

As with any ectopic gestation, treatment options are dependent on whether the patient is clinically stable and can be divided into conservative medical, conservative surgical, or major surgical interventions. Uterine artery embolization and other interventional radiology treatments can be extremely useful particularly when done preoperatively. Injection techniques have been described for successful treatment of small, solid, and nonviable gestations. These are often done in combination and include IM methotrexate, potassium chloride fetal intracardiac injection, and/or

methotrexate injected into the gestational sac in cases with no visible fetal pole or cardiac activity.[20] Conservative surgical techniques include laparoscopic removal, laparoscopic wedge resection, hysteroscopic loop excision, and limited suction curettage for removal of the gestation. In addition to preoperative uterine artery embolization, injection of vasopressin around the gestation can also be useful in decreasing bleeding. In patients who are unstable or are not suitable candidates for conservative management, hysterectomy provides definitive surgical treatment.

REFERENCES

1. Rohilla M, Joshi B, Jain V, Neetimala, Gainder S. Advanced abdominal pregnancy: a search for consensus. Review of literature along with case report. *Arch Gynecol Obstet.* 2018;298(1):1–8.
2. Hailu FG, Yihunie GT, Essa AA, Tsega WK. Advanced abdominal pregnancy, with live fetus and severe preeclampsia, case report. *BMC Pregnancy and Childbirth.* 2017;17(1):243.
3. Bertrand G, Le Ray C, Simard-Emond L, Dubois J, Leduc L. Imaging in the management of abdominal pregnancy: a case report and review of the literature. *J Obstet Gynaecol Can.* 2009;31(1):57–62.
4. Mutarambirwa HD, Kenfack B, Fouogue JT. Term abdominal pregnancy revealed by amnioperitoneum in rural area. *Case Rep Obstet Gynecol.* 2017;2017:4096783.
5. Kunwar S, Khan T, Srivastava K. Abdominal pregnancy: methods of hemorrhage control. *Intractable & rare diseases research.* 2015;4(2):105–107.
6. Marcellin L, Menard S, Lamau MC, et al. Conservative management of an advanced abdominal pregnancy at 22 weeks. *AJP reports.* 2014;4(1):55–60.
7. Cardosi RJ, Nackley AC, Londono J, Hoffman MS. Embolization for advanced abdominal pregnancy with a retained placenta. A case report. *J Reprod Med.* 2002;47(10):861–863.
8. Timor-Tritsch IE, Khatib N, Monteagudo A, Ramos J, Berg R, Kovacs S. Cesarean scar pregnancies: experience of 60 cases. *J Ultrasound Med.* 2015;34(4):601–610.
9. Cali G, Forlani F, Timor-Tritsch IE, Palacios-Jaraquemada J, Minneci G, D'Antonio F. Natural history of Cesarean scar pregnancy on prenatal ultrasound: the crossover sign. *Ultrasound Obstet Gynecol.* 2017;50(1):100–104.
10. Gonzalez N, Tulandi T. Cesarean scar pregnancy: a systematic review. *J Minim Invasive Gynecol.* 2017;24(5):731–738.
11. Cali G, Timor-Tritsch IE, Palacios-Jaraquemada J, et al. Outcome of Cesarean scar pregnancy managed expectantly: systematic review and meta-analysis. *Ultrasound Obstet Gynecol.* 2018;51(2):169–175.
12. Timor-Tritsch IE, Monteagudo A, Cali G, et al. Cesarean scar pregnancy and early placenta accreta share common histology. *Ultrasound Obstet Gynecol.* 2014;43(4):383–395.
13. Cahill AG, Beigi R, Heine RP, Silver RM, Wax JR. Placenta accreta spectrum. *Am J Obstet Gynecol.* 2018;219(6): B2–b16.

14. Kirk E, Condous G, Haider Z, Syed A, Ojha K, Bourne T. The conservative management of cervical ectopic pregnancies. *Ultrasound Obstet Gynecol.* 2006;27(4): 430−437.

15. Monteagudo A, Minior VK, Stephenson C, Monda S, Timor-Tritsch IE. Non-surgical management of live ectopic pregnancy with ultrasound-guided local injection: a case series. *Ultrasound Obstet Gynecol.* 2005;25(3):282−288.

16. Fylstra DL. Cervical pregnancy: 13 cases treated with suction curettage and balloon tamponade. *Am J Obstet Gynecol.* 2014;210(6):581 e1−5.

17. Wang Y, Xu B, Dai S, Zhang Y, Duan Y, Sun C. An efficient conservative treatment modality for cervical pregnancy: angiographic uterine artery embolization followed by immediate curettage. *Am J Obstet Gynecol.* 2011;204(1): 31 e1−7.

18. Larrain D, Marengo F, Bourdel N, et al. Proximal ectopic pregnancy: a descriptive general population-based study and results of different management options in 86 cases. *Fertil Steril.* 2011;95(3):867−871.

19. Ackerman TE, Levi CS, Dashefsky SM, Holt SC, Lindsay DJ. Interstitial line: sonographic finding in interstitial (cornual) ectopic pregnancy. *Radiology.* 1993;189(1): 83−87.

20. Timor-Tritsch IE, Monteagudo A, Lerner JP. A 'potentially safer' route for puncture and injection of cornual ectopic pregnancies. *Ultrasound Obstet Gynecol.* 1996;7(5): 353−355.

Advanced Gestation in a Challenging Location Simulation

MATERIALS NEEDED
- Volunteer to act as standardized patient
- Paper and pencil

KEY PERSONNEL
- Attending obstetrician
- Maternal−fetal medicine specialist
- Anesthesiologist
- Surgical specialties (as available for your institution)
- Neonatologist
- Resident physician (if available in your institution)
- Nurse

SAMPLE SCENARIO
Patient is a 24-year-old G3P2002 at 28 weeks gestation based on last menstrual period who presents with abdominal pain. Patient has not had any prenatal care. On exam, fetal parts are easily palpable under the patient's skin. Sonogram shows a fetus in the abdomen with no surrounding myometrium. Convene an interdisciplinary team and develop a plan for management of this patient.

DEBRIEFING AND DOCUMENTATION
- Review key team members to involve in planning
- Discuss the following aspects of delivery
  - Location
  - Timing
  - Surgical technique
  - Safety measures
- Communicate with patient and family

Simulation Checklist		Time	Comments
Specialists invited to interdisciplinary meeting	Obstetrics		
	Maternal–fetal medicine		
	Anesthesia		
	Surgical specialties		
	Urology		
	Critical care		
	Interventional radiology		
	Neonatology		
	Nursing		
Logistic considerations	Location of delivery		
	Timing of delivery		
Prematurity considerations	Antenatal steroids		
	Magnesium sulfate		
Surgical preparation	Vascular access		
	Availability of blood products		
	Placement of ureteral stents		
Surgical considerations	Type of incision		
	Planned surgical procedure		
	Techniques to minimize blood loss		
Communication	Opinions of all specialties valued		
	Communicated risks, benefits of each approach with patient		
	Shared decision making with patient valued		

Technical Skills	Non-Technical Skills
Laparotomy approach	Communication with team members
Performance of hysterectomy	Interdisciplinary planning
Performance of uterine artery ligation	Task management
Performance of hypogastric artery ligation	Teamwork

Let's debrief. . .

Technical and non-technical skills for complex surgical case

Appendix A

LIST OF ABBREVIATIONS

AAO × 3	Awake, alert, and oriented to person, place, and time
ABC	Airway, breathing, and circulation
ACOG	The American Congress of Obstetricians and Gynecologists
ACLS	Advanced cardiac life support
AED	Automated external defibrillator
ALARA	As low as reasonably achievable
AFE	Amniotic fluid embolism
APGAR	Appearance, pulse, grimace, activity, respiration
APH	Antepartum hemorrhage
aPTT	Activated partial thromboplastin time
AST	Aspartate aminotransferase
BiPAP	Bilevel positive airway pressure
BP	Blood pressure
BPM	Beats per minute
Ca	Calcium
CBC	Complete blood count
Cc	Cubic centimeter
CHTN	Chronic hypertension
CO_2	Carbon dioxide
CPAP	Continuous positive airway pressure
CPR	Cardiopulmonary resuscitation
CT	Computerized tomography
CVA	Cerebrovascular accident
CVP	Central venous pressure
DIC	Disseminated intravascular coagulation
DM	Diabetes mellitus
ECG or EKG	Electrocardiogram
ECV	External cephalic version
EFM	Electronic fetal monitoring
ET	Endotracheal
EMS	Emergency medical services
FiO_2	Fraction of inspired oxygen
FFP	Fresh frozen plasma
FHR	Fetal heart rate
HCT	Hematocrit
HELLP syndrome	Hemolysis, elevated liver enzymes, and low platelets syndrome
HR	Heart rate
HIV	Human immunodeficiency virus
IM	Intramuscular
J	Joules
LBW	Low birthweight
LMA	Laryngeal mask airway
LFT	Liver function test
mL	Milliliters
MHZ	Megahertz
MRI	Magnetic resonance imaging
NRP	Neonatal resuscitation program
PDPH	Postdural puncture headache
PEEP	Positive end-expiratory pressure
PPV	Positive pressure ventilation
SBAR	Situation, background, assessment, recommendations
SMFM	Society for maternal–fetal medicine
SpO_2	Oxygen saturation
TOLAC	Trial of labor after cesarean delivery
VBAC	Vaginal birth after cesarean delivery
VLWB	Very low birth weight

Appendix B

BASIC SIMULATION MATERIALS

A simulation center can be as simple as a doll and a pelvis (Fig. B.1) or as complicated as a high-fidelity simulation center. It is available at our institution (Fig. B.2). Obstetric teams should adapt their simulations to the resources available at their institution.

A vaginal birth simulator will increase the realism of simulations and skills drills. Fig. B.3 shows the NOELLE Interactive Childbirth Simulator Model S560 by Gaumard. This simulator allows computerized control of

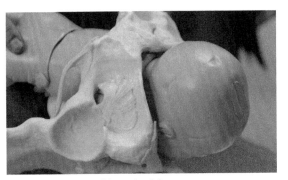

FIG. B.1 Baby manikin and pelvis.

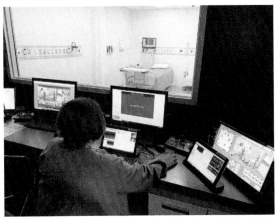

FIG. B.2 Control room at the simulation center UTHSC, Memphis.

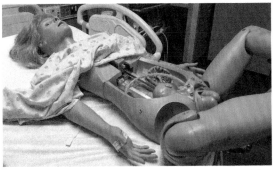

FIG. B.3 NOELLE interactive childbirth simulator model.

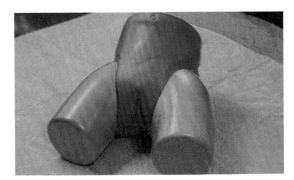

FIG. B.4 PROMPT birthing simulator.

the manikin and realistic simulation of many obstetric emergencies, including shoulder dystocia, breech delivery, eclampsia, and maternal code.

Alternatively, you can purchase a model pelvis and a fetal manikin. This will still allow the team to practice shoulder dystocia and operative vaginal delivery skills. There are a wide variety of prices and degrees of fidelity on the market. Fig. B.4 shows the PROMPT birthing simulator available from Laerdal Medical.

If not using a full-size manikin, a torso manikin can allow the team to practice effective chest compressions, placement of defibrillation pads, and airway management. Fig. B.5 shows the LITTLE JOE Adult CPR Manikin available from Armstrong Medical.

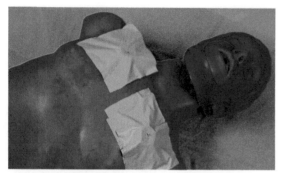
FIG. B.5 Adult CPR manikin.

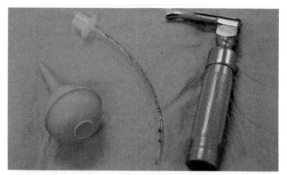
FIG. B.7 Neonatal intubation equipment.

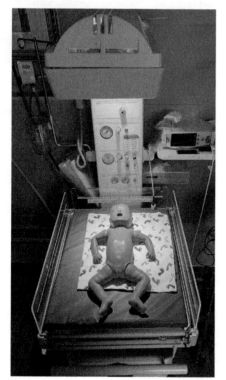
FIG. B.6 Warmer equipment used for neonatal resuscitation.

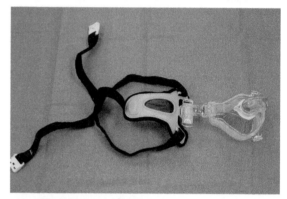
FIG. B.8 Equipment for CPAP.

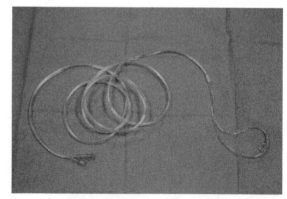
FIG. B.9 Nasal cannula.

For complete multidisciplinary training, set-up should also include a warmer equipment for neonatal resuscitation (Fig. B.6). This can include intubation (Fig. B.7) equipment and a neonatal code cart.

Maternal resuscitation supplies are essential for drills involving maternal cardiac arrest or respiratory distress. These can include CPAP (Fig. B.8), nasal cannula (Fig. B.9), and a maternal code cart (Fig. B.10).

The more hands-on experience your team can get with the actual supplies available on your labor unit, the more realistic their simulation experience will be. Fig. B.11 shows the BAKRI Postpartum Balloon by Cook Medical.

However, to support the realism of the scenario without wasting expensive supplies, laminated images of medications can be substituted for actual medications (Fig. B.12).

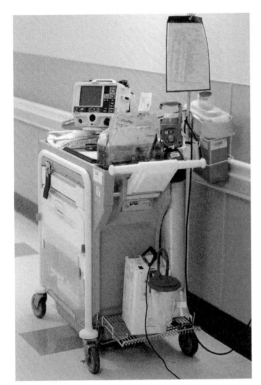

FIG. B.10 Maternal code cart.

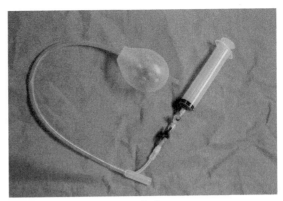

FIG. B.11 Bakri postpartun ballon.

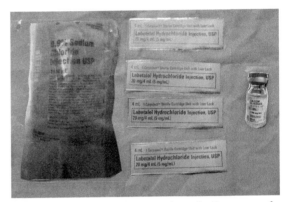

FIG. B.12 Laminates images of medications uses for simulations.

Index

Note: Page numbers followed by "f" indicate figures, "t" indicate tables and "b" indicate boxes.

Printed and bound by CPI Group (UK) Ltd, Croydon, CR0 4YY

03/10/2024

01040349-0011